# MASTER KETTLEBELL GRIPS

Instantly take your kettlebell training to the next level.

WITH LINKS TO VIDEOS

By Taco Fleur

Cavemantraining.com

It is important to know and understand kettlebell grips for efficiency and being able to work the muscles intended for the exercise in question.

# Master Kettlebell Grips

25+ kettlebell grips written by Taco Fleur, Cavemantraining Certified, IKFF Certified Kettlebell Trainer, Kettlebell Level 1 + 2 Trainer, Kettlebell Sport  Rank 2, Kettlebell Science and Application, CrossFit Level 1 Trainer, Kettlebell Sport IKMF Rank 2, MMA Conditioning Level 1, MMA Fitness Level 1 + 2, Punchfit Trainer and Plyometrics Trainer Certified.

www.cavemantraining.com

CAVEMANTRAINING

Welcome to the ultimate kettlebell grip document, if it's a kettlebell grip, you'll find it in this book which is provided to you by Cavemantraining.

The information provided will instantly take your kettlebell training to the next level.

Version:            V7.0

Last updated:       15/09/18

By:                 Taco Fleur

This kettlebell grip book is provided and sponsored by Cavemantraining.com, home of unconventional training methods and the latest online kettlebell training education.

**Grip**

/grɪp/

verb: grip

A manner of holding something.

There are many different types of kettlebell grips you will need to employ during kettlebell training, following are photos and basic explanations of what each different grip is used for. If you enrolled in one of our free or paid online kettlebell courses you will see these different grips referred to. The online grip course is a pre-requisite to our popular kettlebell clean variation course.

Important: with each grip, there are only one or two exercises listed to get a general idea across, but in most cases, there are many more than those listed.  Grips might differ slightly across kettlebells, as the width of the handle increases with some of the classic kettlebells when the weight goes up.

Along your kettlebell journey you will find that different associations or organizations will use different grips for different exercises, and as long as it works and is safe, there is nothing wrong with it.

For illustration purposes, a competition kettlebell is used, which changes in weight but not in size.

Note that these are not Barbell grips, as the names might be the same, the technique is not.

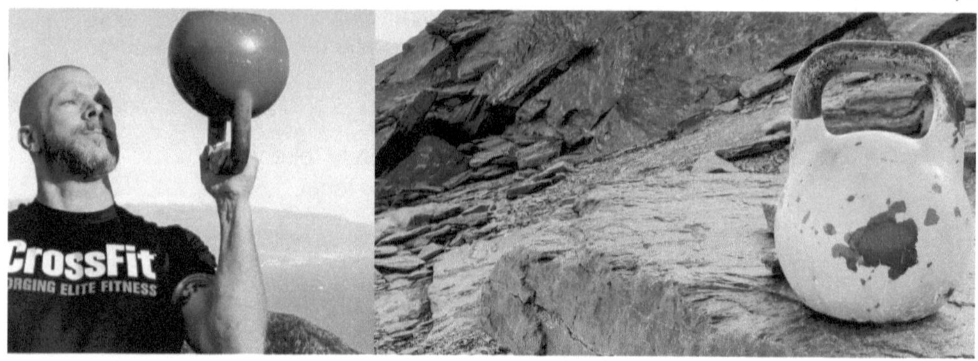

If you have any questions in relation to this document please do not hesitate to post those on our Facebook page, the kettlebell enthusiasts group or the partner that provided you with this document.

**f** /cavemantraining 7,000+

**f** /kettlebelltraining 9,000+

**f** /kettlebell.enthusiasts 3,000+

**f** /kettlebells.for.beginners 300+

Please note that this material may not be reproduced or publicised elsewhere without the written consent of the author me@tacofleur.com.

If this is an electronic copy of the book, please note, this copy is digitally signed and password protected with identifiable information.

All images are copyright © Cavemantraining

Kettlebell stock images are available for purchase or in some cases made available for educational purpose with appropriate credits/links.

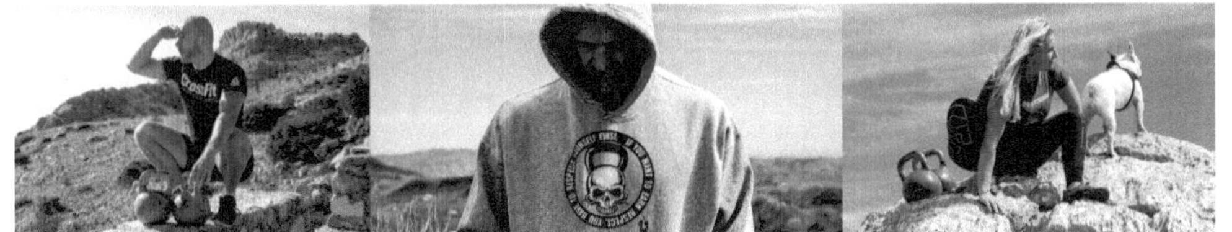

# TABLE OF CONTENTS



You can also chose to enrol in the online course Master Kettlebell Grips and receive your certificate. It's free to take the course!

# PARTNERS AND SPONSORS

www.cavemantraining.com

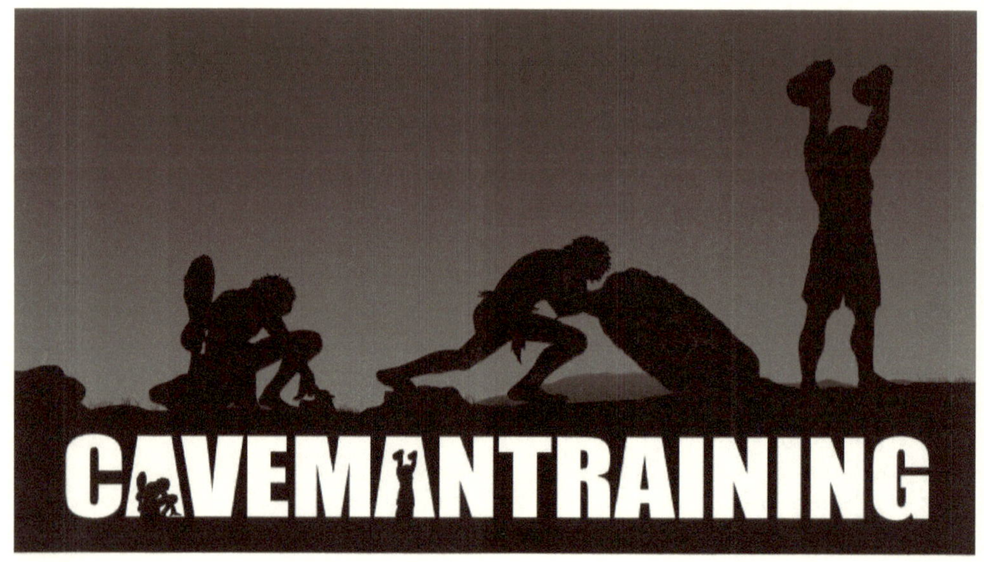


## JOIN OUR GROUP OF KETTLEBELL ENTHUSIASTS

www.facebook.com/groups/kettlebell.enthusiasts/
www.tacofleur.com

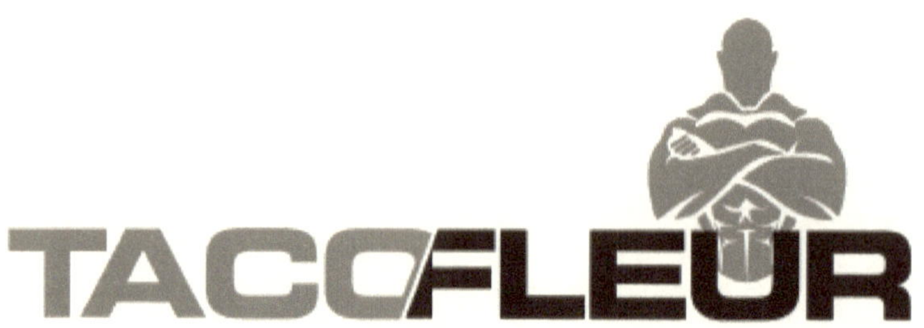

*" excellent document and the content is highly accurate "*

~ Valerie Pawlowski
World Champion Kettlebell Lifting

# General Information

The following rules and tips apply in general to most kettlebell grips. A grip on the kettlebell handle or horns should almost never be tight, it should be as loose as possible without losing grip of the kettlebell and conserving as much grip strength without burning out the muscles.

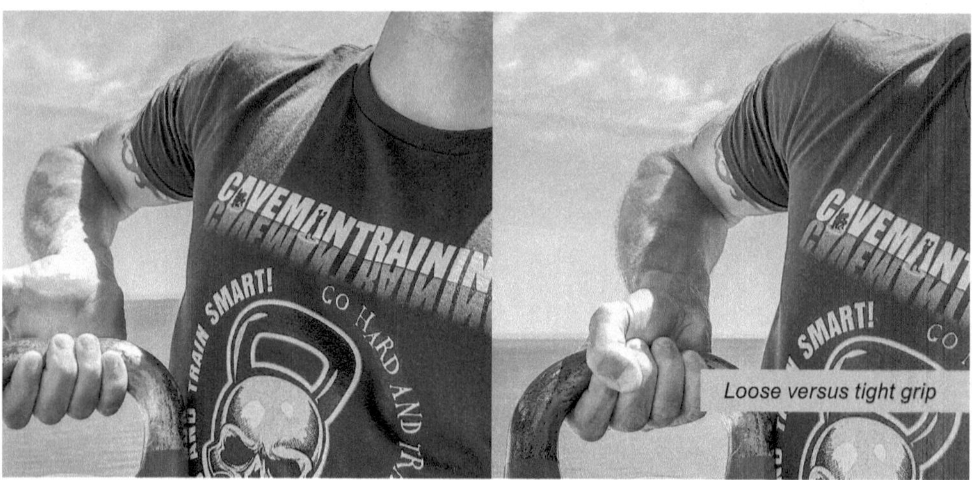

*Loose versus tight grip*

**Blisters** usually occur when the skin is folded within the grip, especially when using heavy weights or doing high volume reps. Try and slide your fingers around the handle or horns while keeping skin folds from occurring and then close the grip. Another cause for blisters is friction, avoid friction by proper kettlebell guidance (which you'll learn in our courses).

**Ripped** calluses usually occur when there is friction within the palms, biggest culprit is kettlebell bobbing, to prevent the kettlebell from bobbing search for my article online 'kettlebell swing insert', the insert prevents the kettlebell from doing a full pendulum which is usually causing abrupt stopping of the kettlebell.

> " You should look at it like this. If you're making the pendulum movement and let the bell go where it wants to go, it abruptly gets stopped by your body, i.e. your arms hit your thighs or whatever part of the body, the bell will want to keep going, this is creating the friction in your hands, on high reps or heavy weight this will cause blisters.
>
> To fix, think about directing the weight to the back, create a deep insert, think first part of the swing PENDULUM and then bang, INSERT. Direct the weight to the back. Hope that helps. "

The most common grip and transition is that from hook grip to loose grip which occurs during the clean and rack, the hook grip is also used for single arm swings and snatches, the second most common grip is the double hand grip which is used for double arm swings.

This transition is one that beginners should focus on, the need to want to hold the kettlebell handle tight, and perform no transition is high with beginners. This is such an important concept that everyone should spend a lot of time on until they get it right. I can highly recommend performing assisted cleans to work on this, you can see more about this here: www.cavemantraining.com/cavemantraining/day-one/

The above are just a few tips and fundamentals to get you going with your grip on the kettlebell, should you want to learn much more, search the web for *"Kettlebell Training Fundamentals"*, Cavemantraining has books, courses, apps, videos and more out on this topic.

- **Master The Hip Hinge**
  On Amazon, iTunes, or Cavemantraining

- **Master The Lunge**
  On Amazon, iTunes, or Cavemantraining

- **Master Kettlebell Grips**
  This book

- **Kettlebell Training Fundamentals**
  On Amazon, iTunes, or Cavemantraining
  Contains the kettlebell grips and racking book

- **Master The Kettlebell Clean**
  On Amazon, iTunes, or Cavemantraining

- **Master The Kettlebell Press**
  On Amazon or Cavemantraining

- **Master The Kettlebell Swing**
  On Amazon or Cavemantraining

- **Snatch Physics**
  On Amazon or Cavemantraining

- **Kettlebell Workouts And Challenges 1.0**
  On Amazon, iTunes, or Cavemantraining

- **Flexibility, Mobility, and Strength Without Yoga**
  On Amazon, iTunes, or Cavemantraining

- **Android Apps**
  https://play.google.com/store/apps/dev?id=8257172044033882048

- **YouTube videos**
  https://www.youtube.com/Cavemantraining

- **And more on Cavemantraining**

# Why should you learn about grips?

It is important to know and understand kettlebell grips for efficiency and being able to work the muscles intended for the exercise in question. Employing an incorrect grip can mean pain; being uncomfortable; cause for injury; exhausting grip, forearm, biceps or shoulder muscles and losing focus on the muscles targeted with a specific exercise.

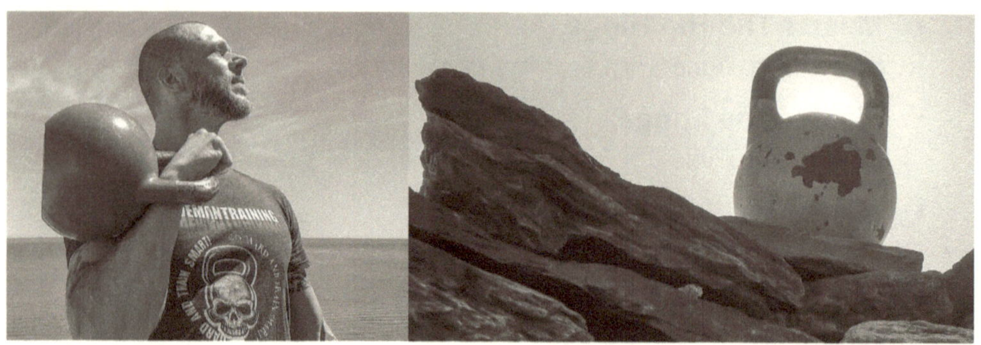

# Why use different grips?

If you're asking this question, then you're asking the right question because knowing a lot of grips is cool, but knowing why you would change grip or use one over the other is even  cooler and the part you should really understand.

During kettlebell training, you employ different grips to make certain exercises more efficient, but you also change grips to increase difficulty and challenge other muscle groups. Sometimes when your training gets stale you might even employ a different grip to please the mind.

While knowing kettlebell grips and when to employ them is important and one of the kettlebell fundamentals, the second most important thing you should start looking into is racking a kettlebell. It might seem insignificant, but a lot hinges on how you rack your kettlebell, in fact, some people give up on kettlebell training because they can't get comfortable in the racking position or can't find the proper position for the bell to rest.

*Search Google for '**Cavemantraining Kettlebell Racking**'
to start learning about this next topic in kettlebell fundamentals.*

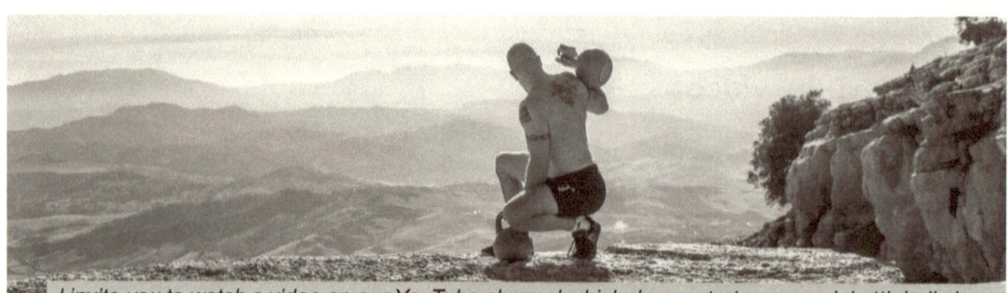

*I invite you to watch a video on our YouTube channel which demonstrates several  kettlebell clean transitions into different grips https://youtu.be/ApbEAUy2Tbo*

# 45-Degree Angle

In grips employed for racking or pressing, the handle should be positioned at a 45-degree angle within the palm, one corner positioned between the thumb and index finger, and the other corner being past the heel of the palm. The reason for this position is to keep the wrist straight and hand in line with the forearm, this will avoid pressure on the wrist. A bent wrist means there is a kink in the line through which power will be lost during pressing plus cause for potential injury.

When working with a light kettlebell this might not be so noticeable, but when working with heavier kettlebells the pressure can be enormous, cause damage to the wrist and/or prevent you from being able to press the kettlebell up.

When people first start training with a kettlebell, you'll find that they employ the broken wrist grip to relieve the pressure that the bell provides on the forearm, this is especially so for new people who are not used to this pressure. You should take the person aside and have them play with the grip, handle position and bell positioning until they feel ok with the pressure of the kettlebell being in the correct position. You should also explain that it's quite normal to experience some mild discomfort until the area is more conditioned.

*See illustrations below for correct 45-degree handle angle in the palm.*

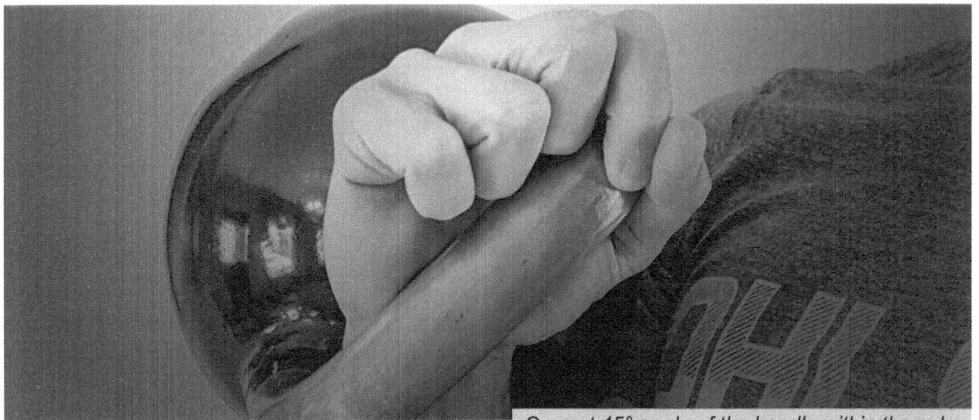

*Correct 45° angle of the handle within the palm*

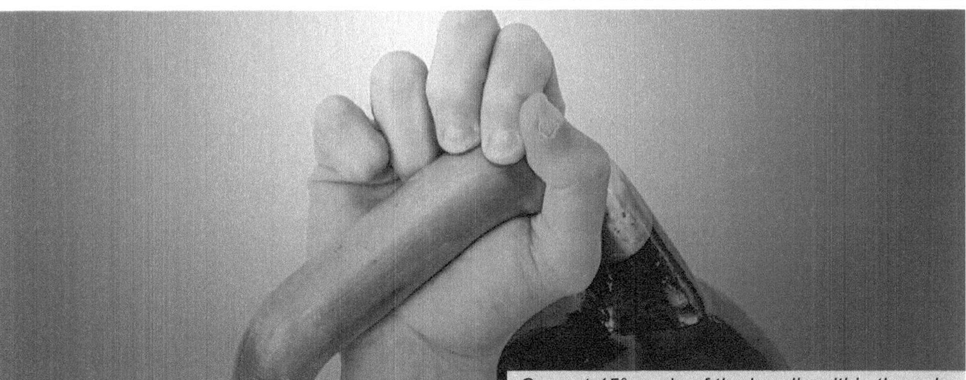

*Correct 45° angle of the handle within the palm*

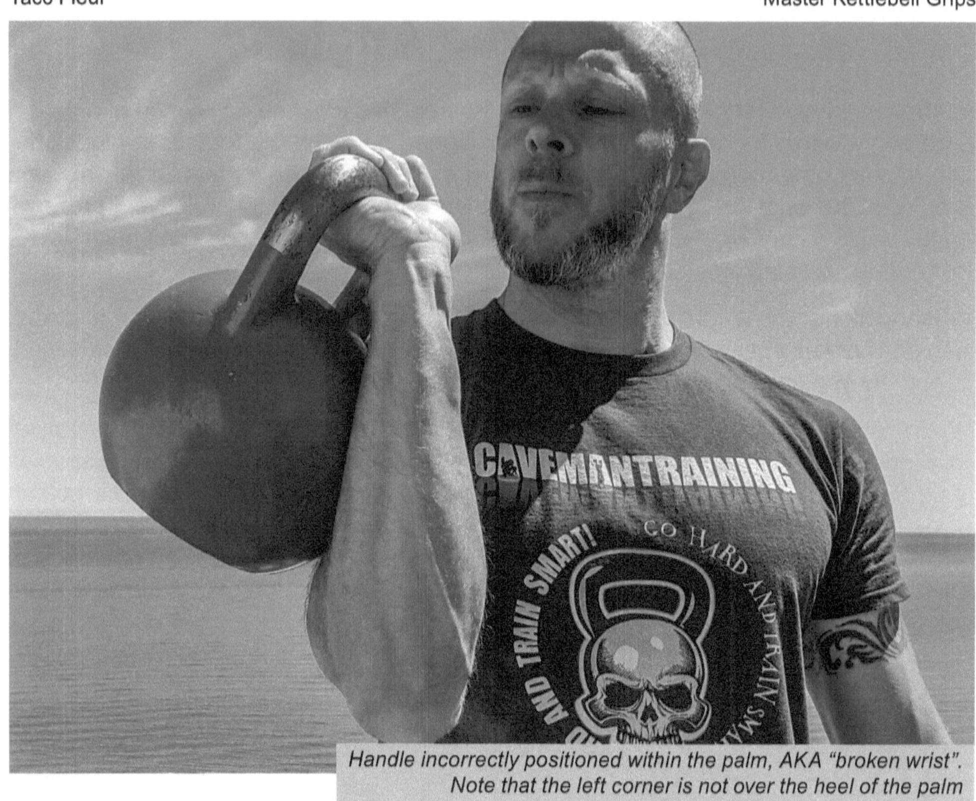

Handle incorrectly positioned within the palm, AKA "broken wrist".
Note that the left corner is not over the heel of the palm

# Anatomy Of The Kettlebell

Following illustration breaks down the anatomy of the kettlebell, knowing the exact names for parts of the kettlebell will help you understand given instructions better and/or increase clarity when teaching kettlebell training.

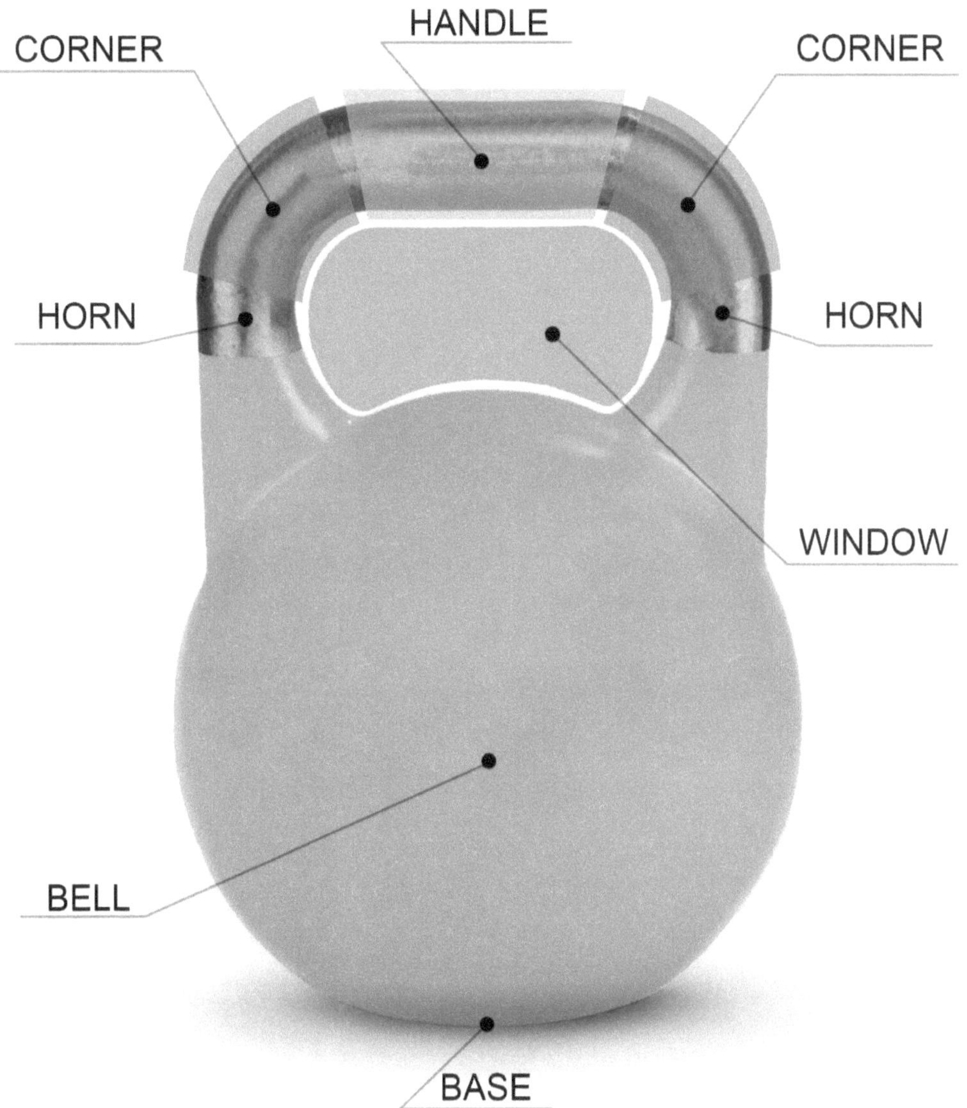

# Grip Categories

Grips can be categorized in the following categories:

- Pressing grips
- Racking grips
- Lifting grips
- Ballistic grips
- Juggling grips

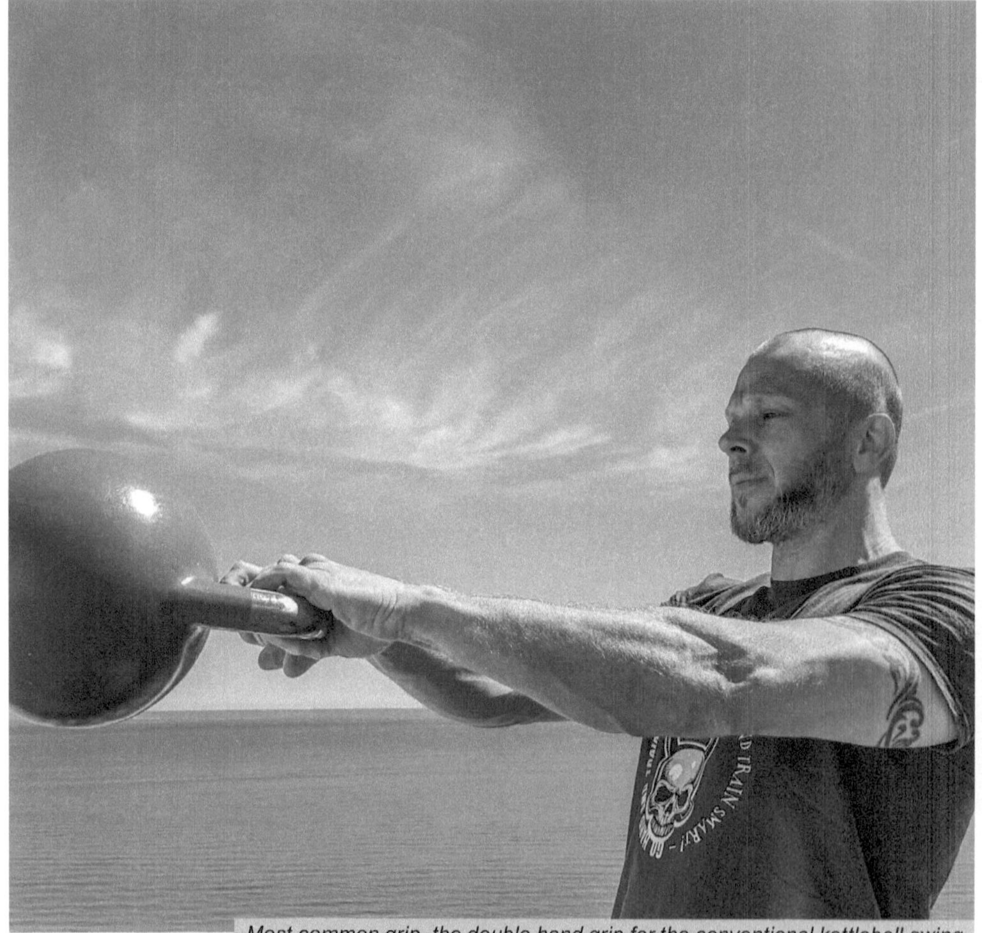

*Most common grip, the double hand grip for the conventional kettlebell swing*

# Broken Wrist Grip — incorrect grip

As the name implies, this is not a grip you'll want to employ. It's named such because the straight line your arm and palm should be in is broken. A correct kettlebell grip is one of the main things to focus on when you start kettlebell training. You have to get it right, take some time away from everyone and take a light kettlebell, play with it, move it around till you find the two or three points in racking where the weight should rest. The resting points are; around the heel of the palm; on the forearm; and against the biceps when in cradle racking position.

When your wrist is not straight/neutral in racking or overhead position, all the weight is pulling down on your wrist. Most people employ this incorrect grip because they might feel less pressure on the forearm, however, one should take the time to find the right resting points to maintain a neutral wrist. The second cause for an incorrect grip/insert is a tight grip and not opening up during the clean for a proper hand insert.

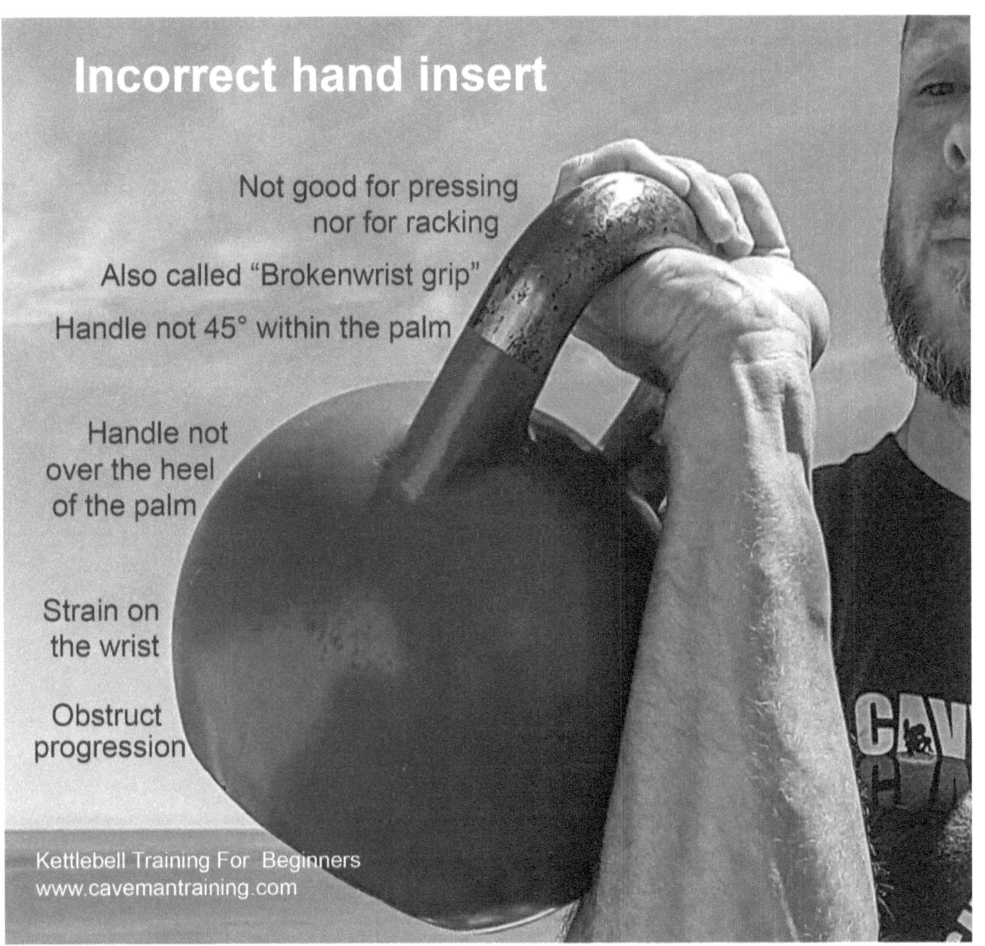

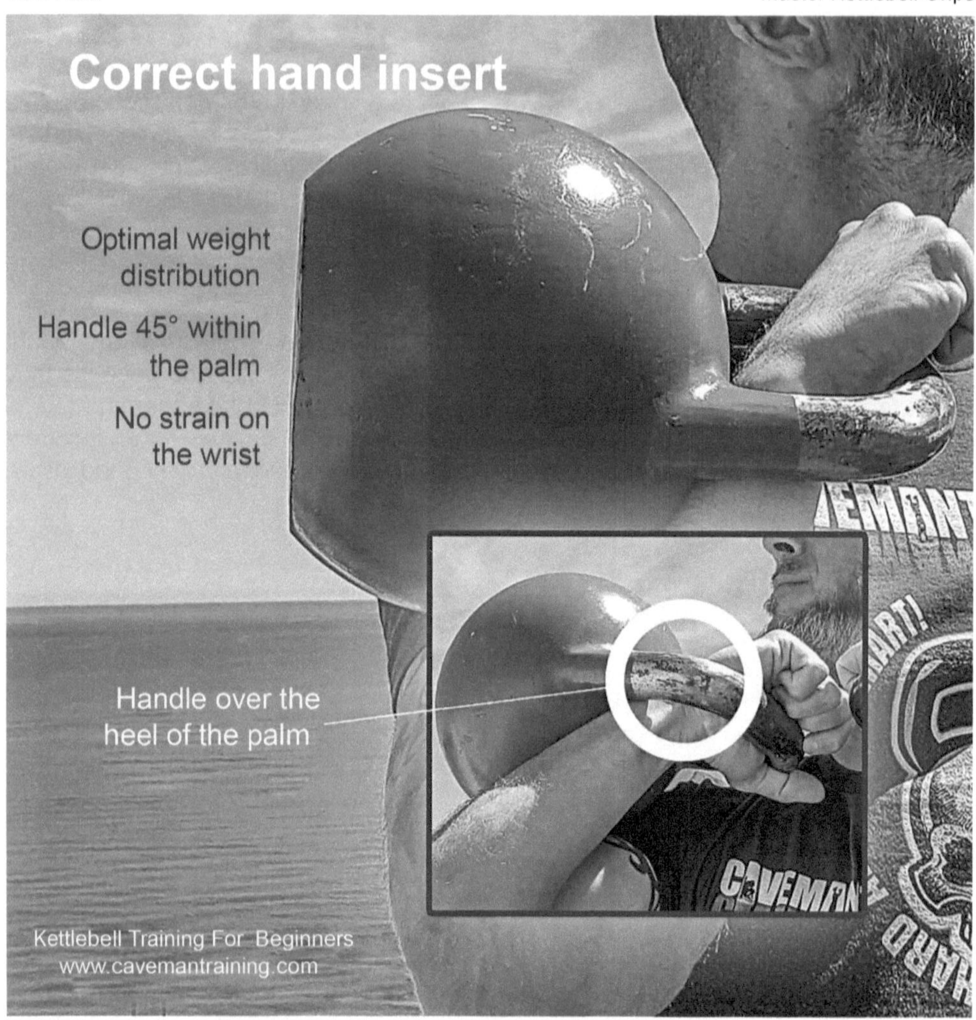


The above photo can be saved/shared from the following link:
www.facebook.com/photo.php?fbid=10154859982094327


The photo below can be saved/shared from:
www.facebook.com/photo.php?fbid=10154859982099327

# Why do competition kettlebells feel heavier?

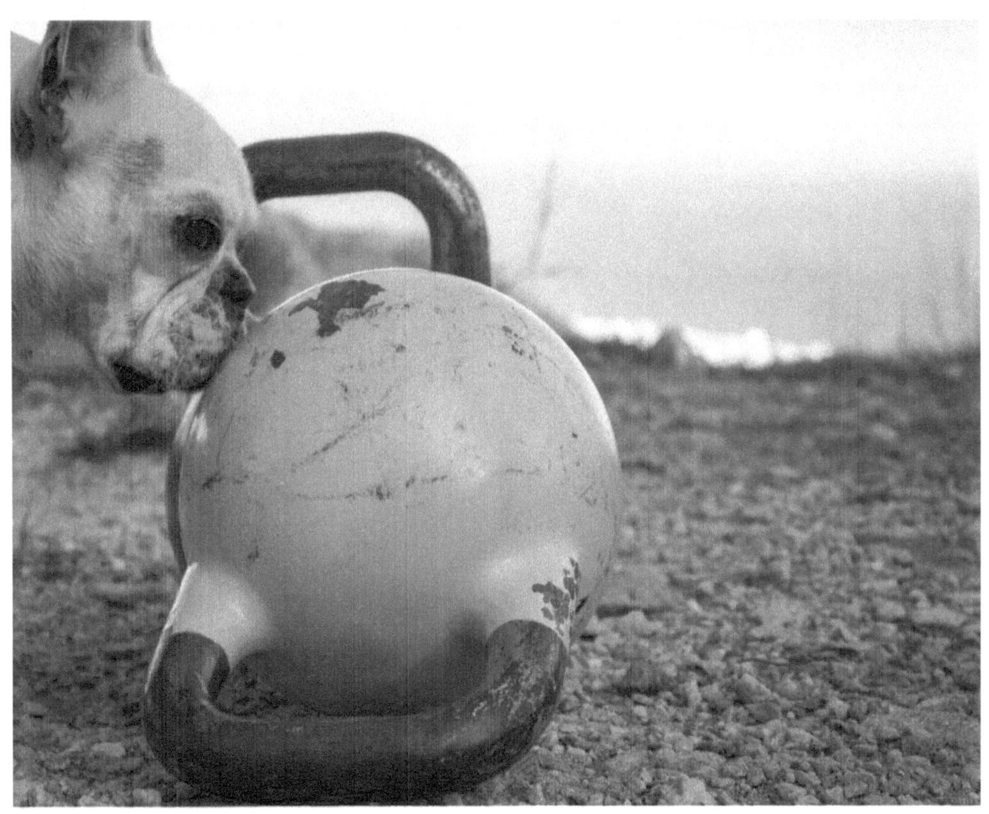

If you have access to competition kettlebells and classic kettlebells (cast iron) you might have noticed that a 32kg (or any other weight) competition kettlebell can feel heavier than a 32kg classic kettlebell, why is that?

Take note that the handle diameter on the competition kettlebells remains pretty much the same no matter what weight, whereas with the classic kettlebells it usually changes. Both have their advantages and disadvantages, depending on how you look at it, and what your goals are.

The larger the diameter of the handle, the easier it is to hold/grip it; this needs to be considered in the context of hand to handle ratio as well. A large diameter handle with a small hand is not optimal.

A smaller handle (the competition bell handle) is harder to grip, hence, feels heavier because the forearms need to work harder to maintain grip.

If you do a lot of pressing with a heavy kettlebell, a wider diameter handle will be easier on the palms of your hands, the wider the diameter, the wider the shared surface pressure is. A small diameter handle puts more pressure on the palm as the shared surface pressure is smaller.

Without further ado,
let's dive deep
into the kettlebell grips

# Double Hand Grip

**Grip:** two hands, four fingers closed around the handle placed on the corners or horns depending on hand size and thumbs loose.

**Ideal for:** double-arm swings and deadlifts.

This grip is mostly used for doing double arm swings and deadlifts. Like with most grips, do not turn this into a tight grip, keep some space for the handle to move freely without causing friction. This grip should loosen up at the top part of the swing to stop the grip from burning out. You will have eight fingers around the handle, with big hands your fingers might feel squashed when doing high volume reps, pay particular attention to the ring fingers at high volume reps as they'll be prone to blisters.

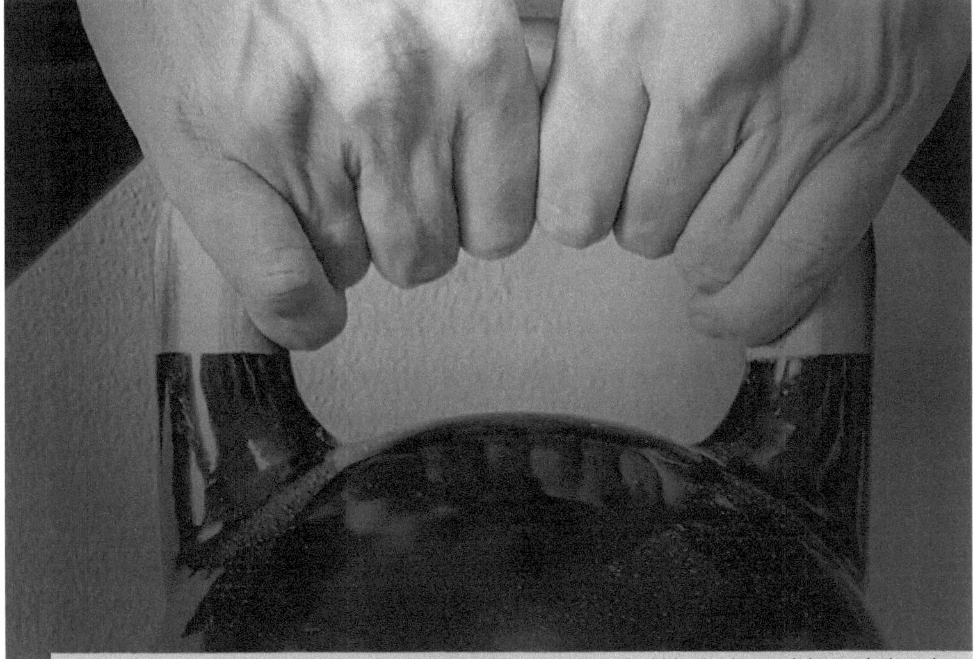

*The grip can be employed with both of the pinkies positioned within the horns (pictured above) or over the horns (pictured further below under the Closed Double Hand Grip).*

# Following
# two grips
# are provided
## by **Valerie Pawlowski**
### World Champion Kettlebell Lifting

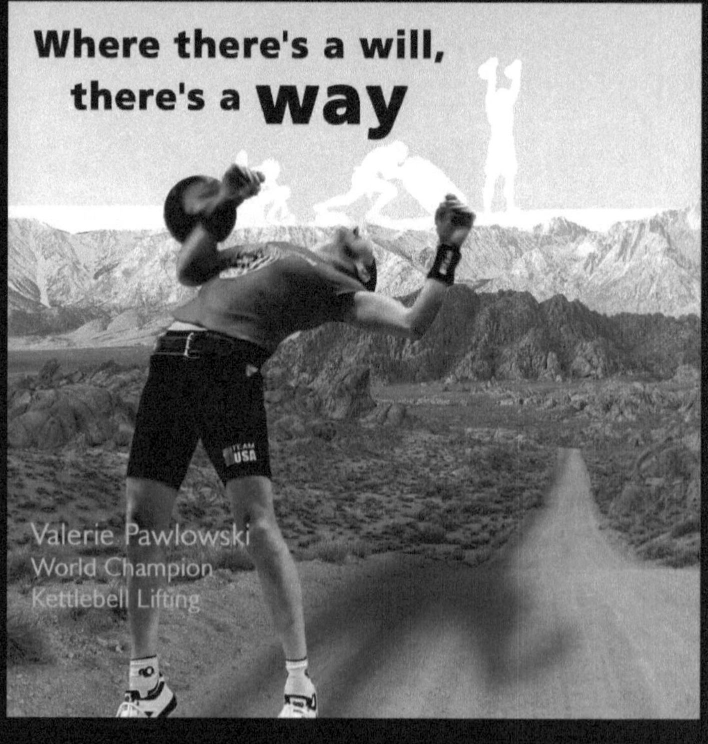

# Swan Grip

This grip is used primarily in rowing drills and pulling or front holding movements.

Grasping with fingers mostly straight in a beak like hold over top of kettlebell with arm bent at wrist and elbow in "S" like position, as that of swan neck, with emphasis on squeeze of fingers and strong forearm engagement this grip works tremendous grip strength for massive finger and forearm recruitment.

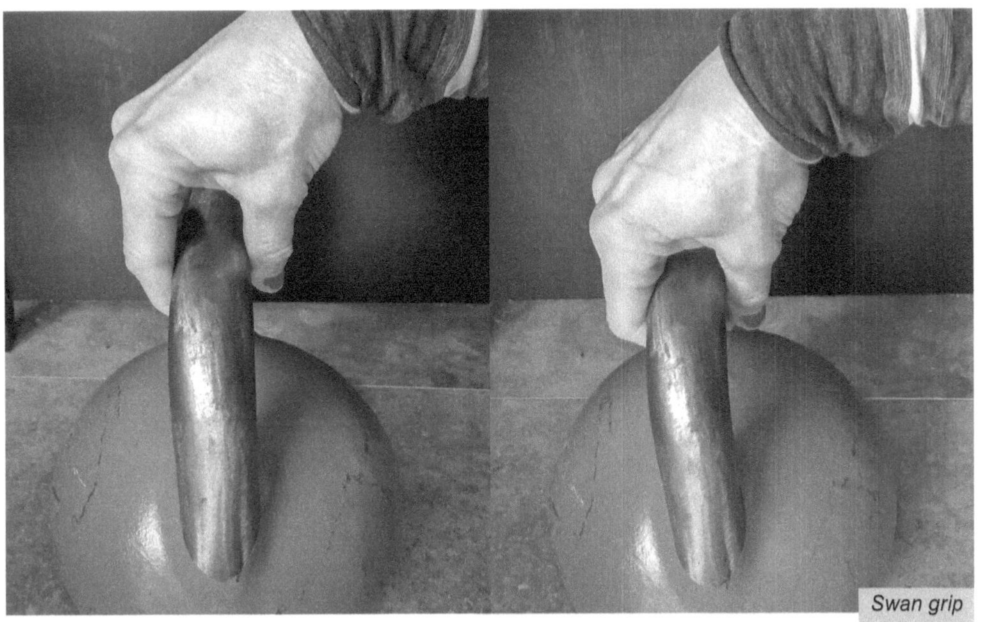

Swan grip

# OK Grip (AKA 2 or 3 Finger Grip)

With thumb and first finger (and middle for 3) in an 2 finger lock wrap around handle. Remaining 3 fingers are off or relaxed (2 off on the ok 3 hold) away from handle.

Useful for carries, swings, clean or row. The thumb and first finger are the most important to primary grip strength. Working with these variations puts attention on the longer lasting strength to hang on to the fullest extent especially digging out on final Snatches.

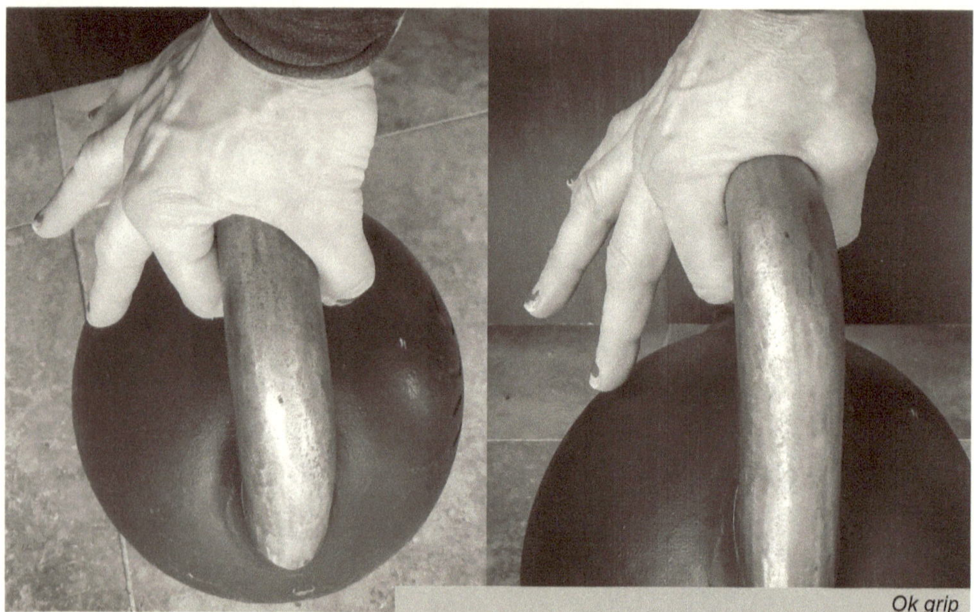

*Ok grip*
*Thanks to Valerie Pawlowski for the photos and information*

# Double Hand Corkscrew Grip

**Grip:** same as the double hand grip but with the horns between the pinkie and ring fingers.

**Ideal for:** double-arm swings and American swings.

This is a grip I've started using when doing heavy high volume swings during the **Caveman Kettlebells 28 Day Swing Challenge**, which I like to call the Double Hand Corkscrew Grip because it's very similar to a grip on a corkscrew, when holding a corkscrew, the screw itself will be positioned between the middle finger and ring finger, but with the kettlebell the horn will be positioned between the ring finger and pinkie. Everything from the Double Hand Grip transfers to this grip. I like to use this grip to switch it up, but also because I have big hands and usually need to put my pinkies over the handles with the Double Hand Grip, with this grip I feel that my fingers are less squashed. It is very important to wrap your pinkies around the horn to prevent them from getting caught in your clothes during the swing. This grip also provides more stability at the top of the American swing and helps prevent skin tears on the outside of the pinkie.

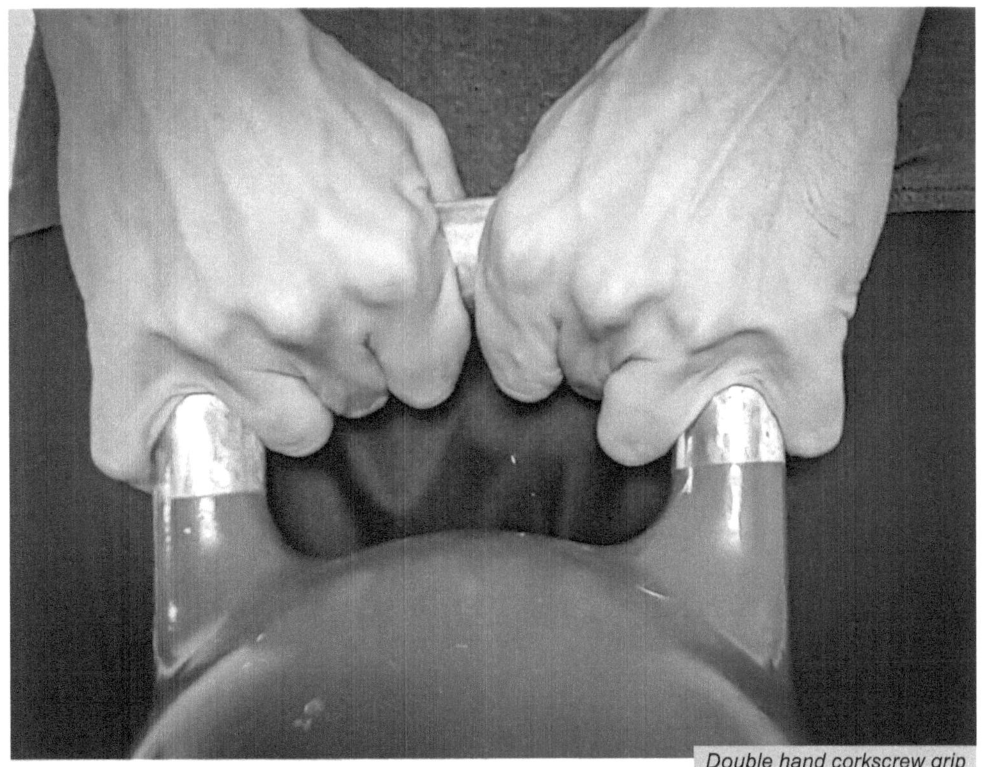

*Double hand corkscrew grip*

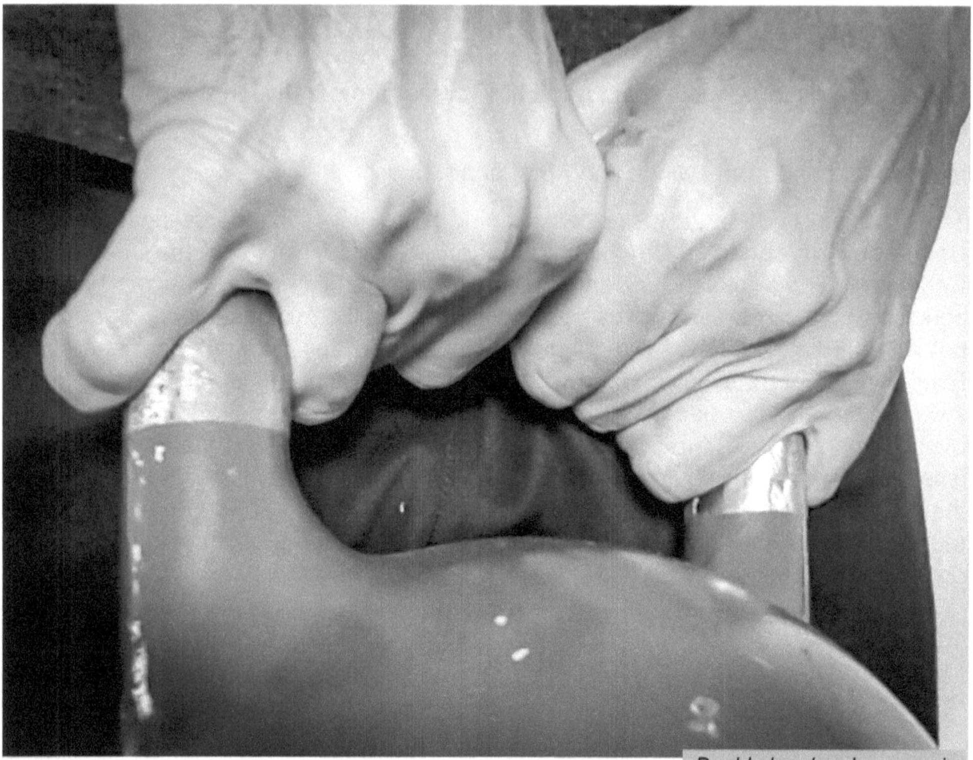

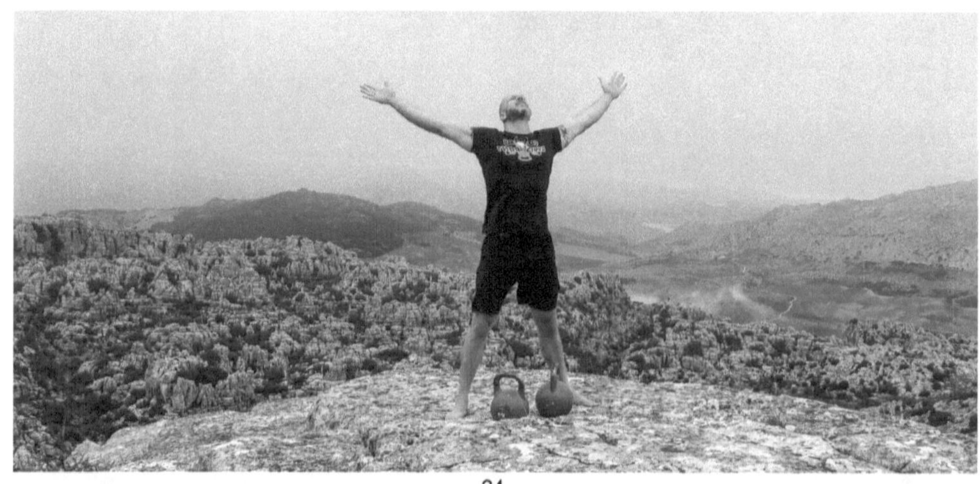

*Double hand corkscrew grip*

# Come and say "hi" on our Facebook

# Closed Double Hand Grip

**Handle:** two hands, four fingers and thumbs locking the index finger down, or locking both the index and middle finger down. Can also be with the pinkies over the horns as illustrated below, in which case it becomes, three fingers plus lock.

**Ideal for:** double-arm swings, deadlifts

Everything from the Double Hand Grip transfers to this grip, the difference is that the thumbs are locking over the index fingers, this grip is for using extremely heavy weights, or high volume swings and the grip is giving up. The lock is also employed to relieve some tension from the forearms. The lock might also be possible with one thumb two fingers. Note: this grip might not be possible with thicker handles.

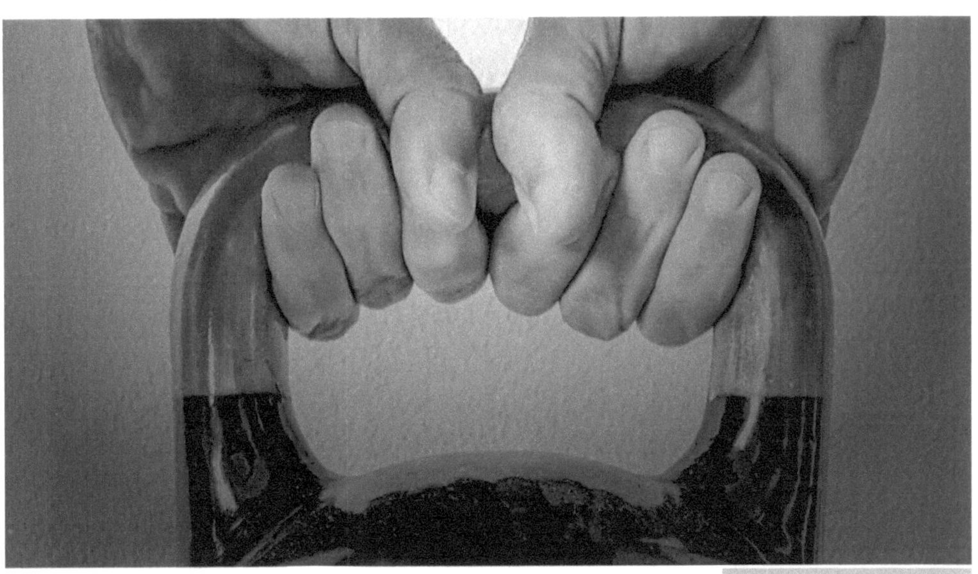

Closed double hand grip

***For online learning please visit the following resources.***

*To learn the Kettlebell Training swing online please visit*
*www.cavemantraining.com*

*For the ebook on the kettlebell training fundamentals please see our publication on amazon.com*

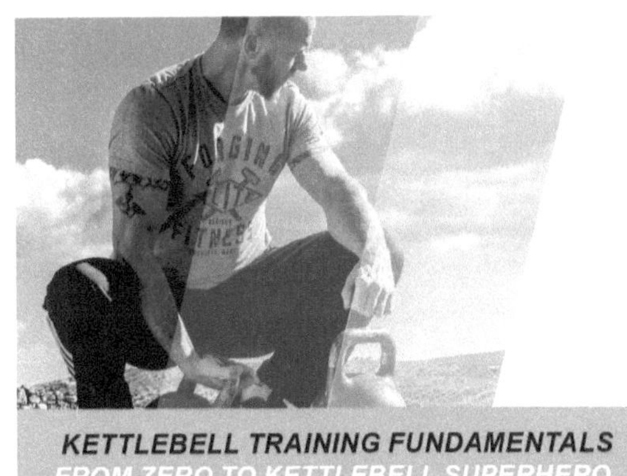

# Hook Grip (AKA Overhand Grip)

**Handle:** one hand, four fingers and thumb loose

**Ideal for:** down-phase of most ballistic movements, dead clean.

With this grip, the handle is positioned within the fingers which are bend, used when the Kettlebell travels downwards for single arm swings and downward phase of snatches. Note that the thumb can move over to the other side of the handle (but not locking finger) and the hand is positioned closer to one side of the handle.

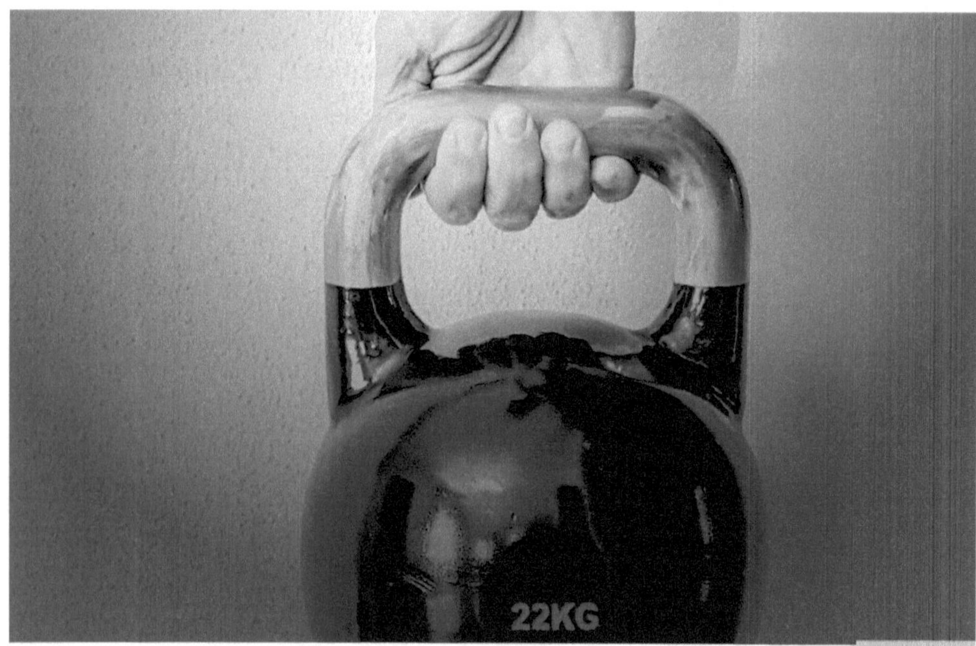

*Hook Grip*

***For online learning please visit the following resources.***

*To learn the Kettlebell Training swing online please visit www.cavemantraining.com*

*For the ebook on the kettlebell training fundamentals please see our publication on amazon.com*

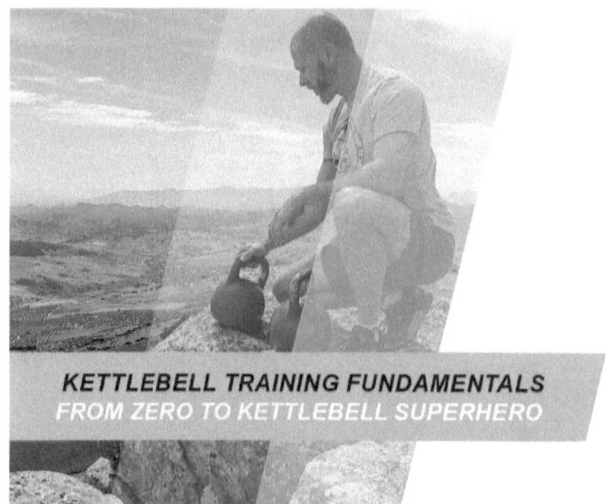

# Closed Hook Grip (AKA C grip)

**Handle:** one hand, four fingers and thumb locking the index finger down, or both the index and middle finger

**Ideal for:** single-arm swings, snatch, dead clean.

This grip is the same as the Hook Grip apart from there being a finger lock with the thumb over forefinger. The lock provides a better grip but also releases tension on the forearms and fingers. If you experience fingers cramps, forearms pains or soreness, try switching to a closed hook grip. Issues arise especially when just starting out with training or when doing high volume reps without implementing a closed grip.

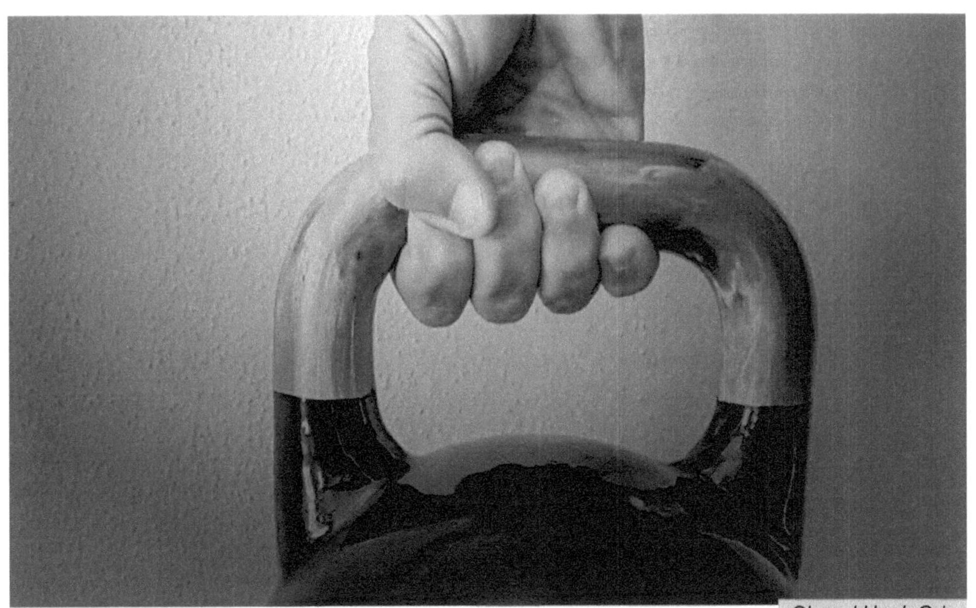

Closed Hook Grip

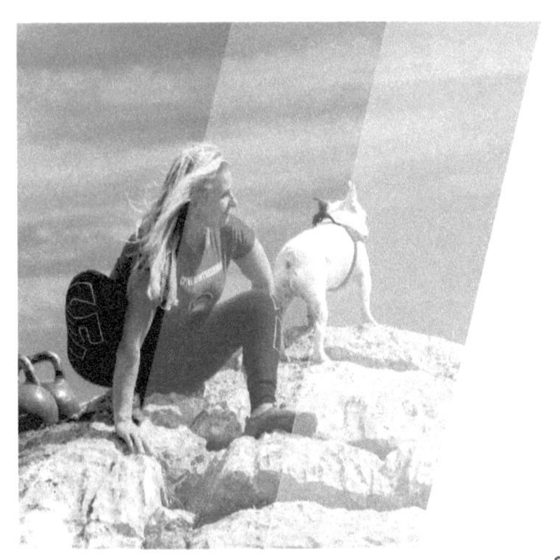

*Become certified online in the kettlebell clean and 70+ variations*

- *Book and videos $29.95*

- *Book, videos, exam, and certificate of participation $39.95*

- *L3.0 Trainer (Become certified) $49.95*

- *L3.1 Trainer (Become certified) $69.95*

www.cavemantraining.com/kettlebell-clean-variations/

# Racking Grip

This is the common grip employed in racking position with a closed but relaxed fist, fingers gently resting on the handle. If you work with two kettlebells you should look at employing the racking safety grip.

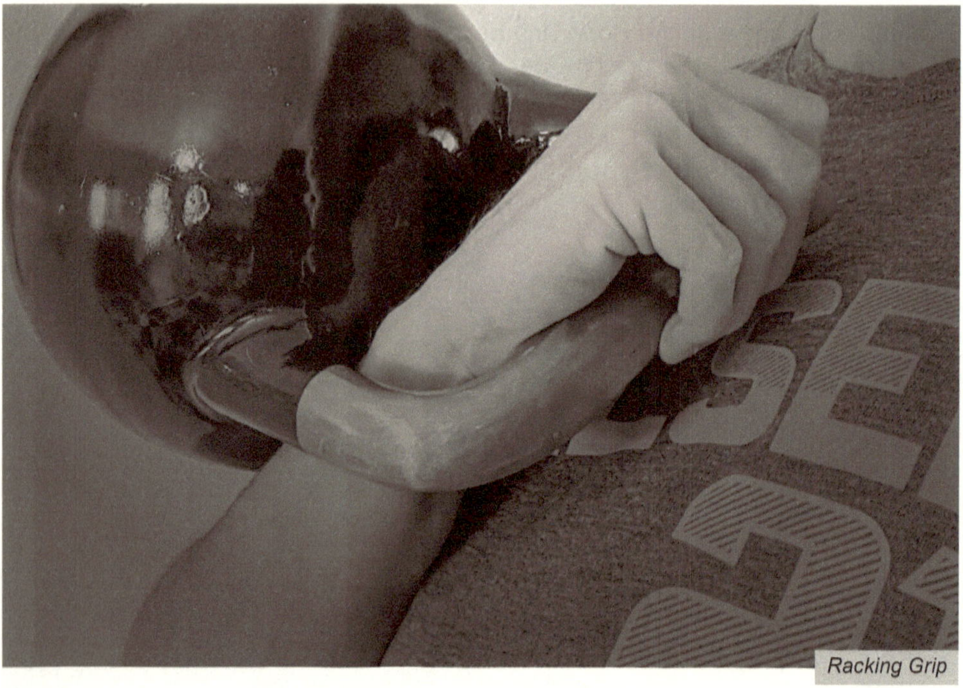

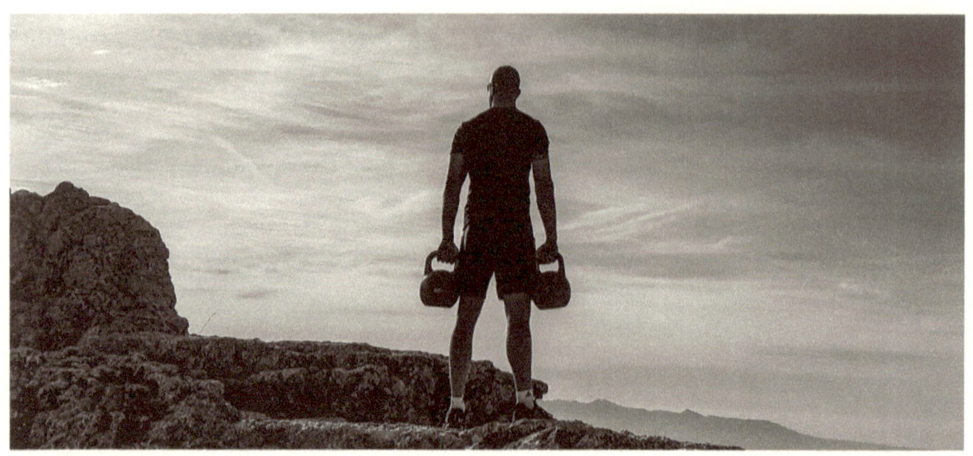

*Racking Grip*

Racking is important for resting, pressing, squatting and all require a different type of rack.

*Search Google for 'Cavemantraining Kettlebell Racking'*
*to get the free info on racking.*

# Racking Safety Grip

With this grip the thumb is over the index finger which are placed over the horn, and the remaining fingers are tucked behind the handle, this grip is used when working with Two kettlebells to protect the fingers from getting caught between the two kettlebell handles.

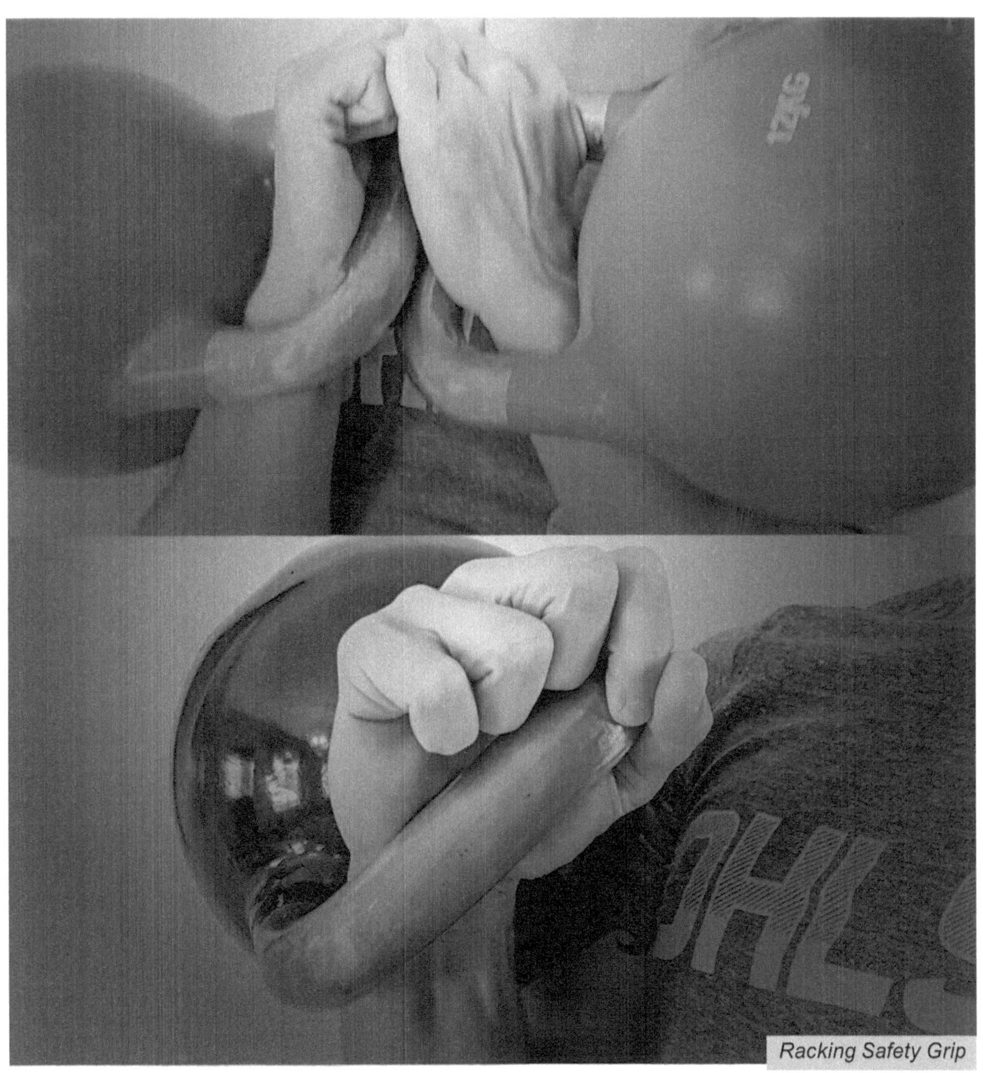

Racking Safety Grip

*Make sure to check out the following article and video  on how to easily find your racking position.*
*10 steps to find your kettlebell racking position easily*

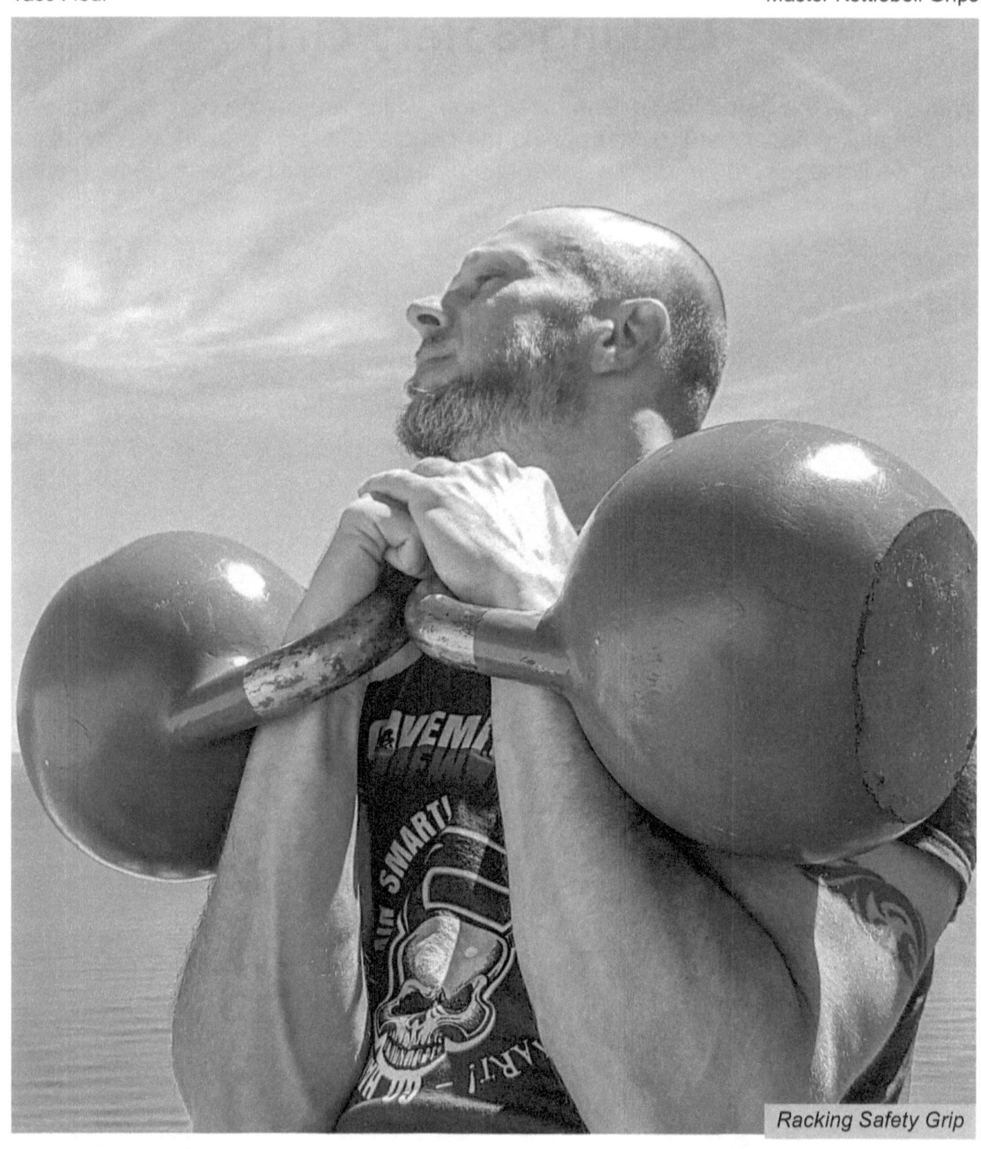

*Racking Safety Grip*

# Flat Hand Grip

The hand is flat or straight with all fingers pointing up and the thumb is around the horn. Can be employed for safety with two kettlebells, racking or in overhead lock-out.

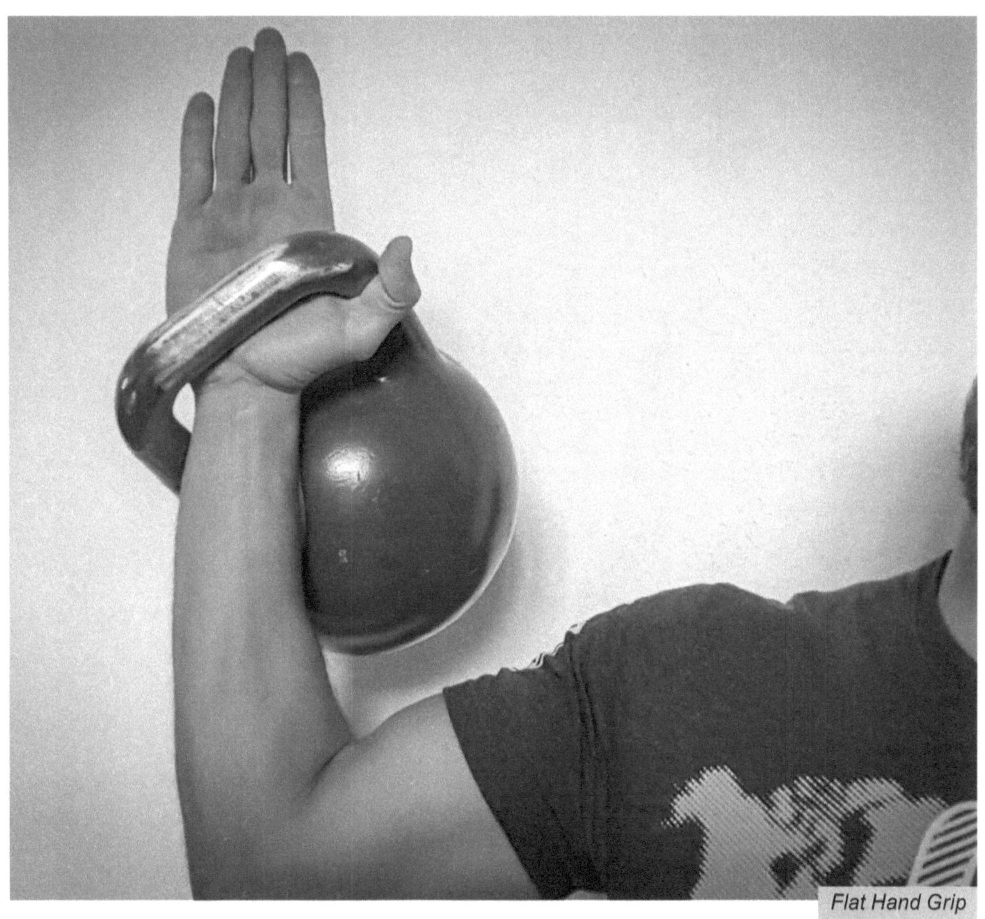

# Pinch Grip

With this grip the thumb and fingers are used to pick up the kettlebell by the base of the kettlebell, this can only be performed with a smaller classic kettlebell. Used for working grip strength.

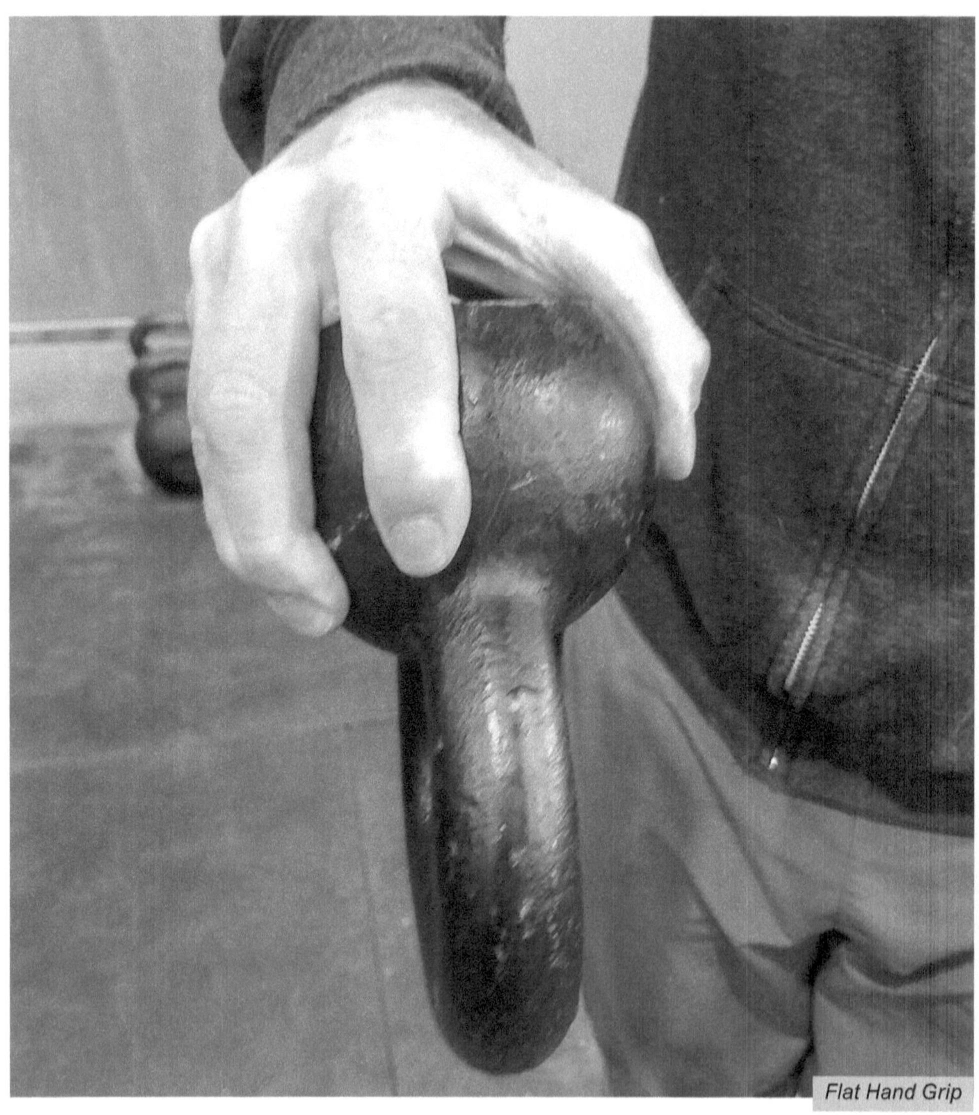

Flat Hand Grip

*Photo provided by Robert Gagnon SFG II*
*www.RobGagnon.com*

# Farmer Grip

**Grip:** middle of the handle.

**Handle:** one hand, four fingers and thumb locking the index finger down, or both the index and middle finger

Ideal for: farmer walks, suitcase dead lifts

With this grip, the hand is placed in the middle of the handle, and used when carrying a heavy Kettlebell beside the body with farmer walks or dead lifts. It should be noted that although the farmer walk grip is usually with a firm grip —contrary to most other grips— you can perform farmer walks with a hook grip as well to challenge the fingers more.

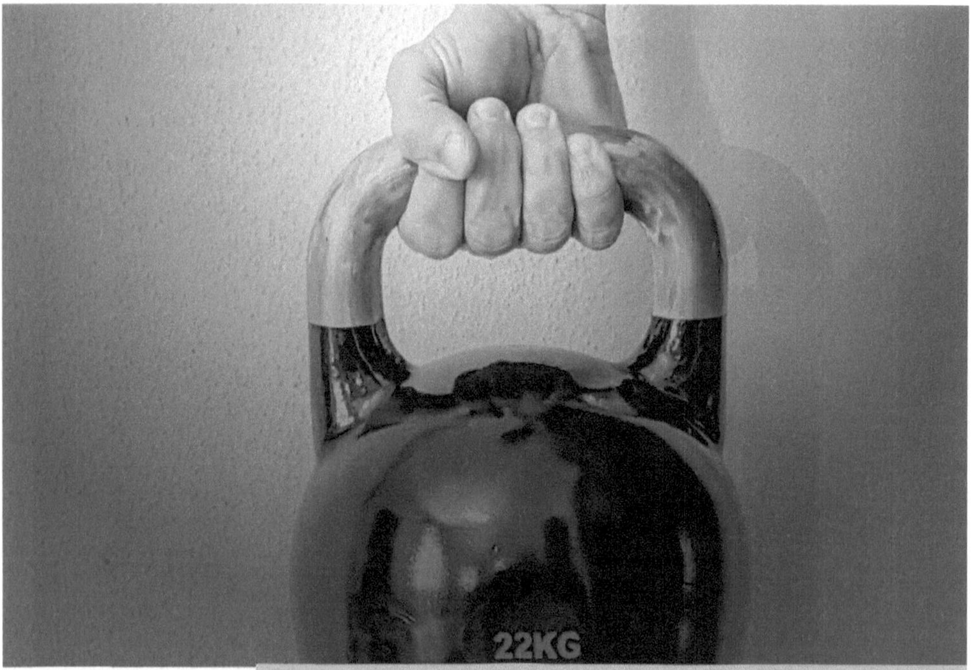

*Farmer walks in action: https://www.youtube.com/watch?v=jqs8NGg50C0*

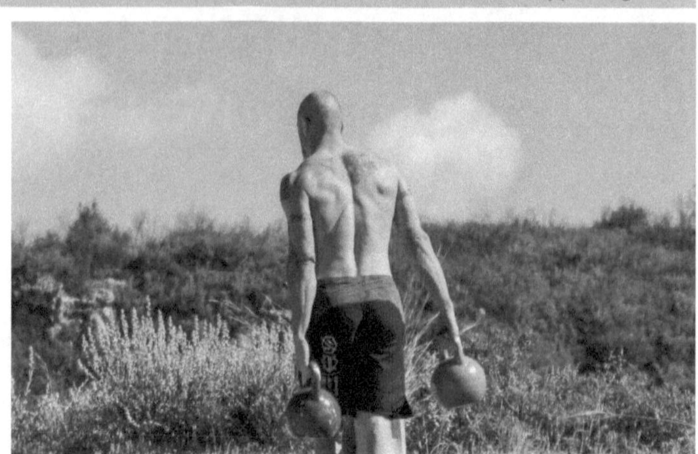

*Farmer walks near Barranco Blanco on the Costa del Sol*

# Tip of the Fingers Grip AKA Gorilla Grip

**Grip:** tip of the fingers.

**Handle:** the handle lays in the tips of the fingers which are shaped like when manicuring the finger nails.

**Ideal for:** farmer walks, suitcase dead lifts, dead lifts.

This grip, is an awesome grip to work on grip strength, I personally started using this to improve my grip strength for BJJ (martial art) and baptised it the Gorilla Grip. The handle should nearly be falling of the fingers that's how little grip should be used. The thumb is not used, just the four finger tips.

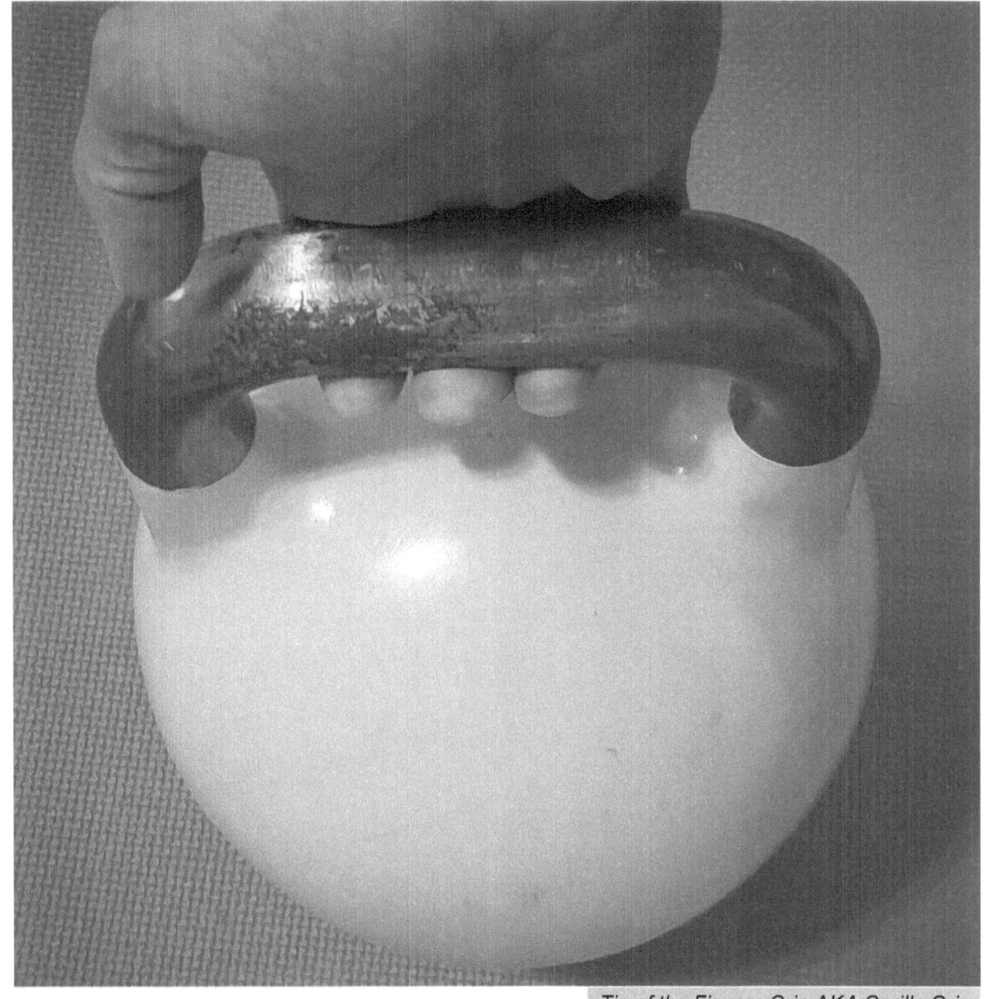

*Tip of the Fingers Grip AKA Gorilla Grip*

# Bottoms Up Grip

**Handle:** one hand, four fingers and thumb crushing the handle

**Ideal for:** bottoms up press, bottoms up squat

This grip is performed with a strong and firm grip on the handle while the Kettlebell is upside down, and used for bottoms up press or bottoms up Turkish get-up. The bottoms-up grip is great to work on grip strength and stability.

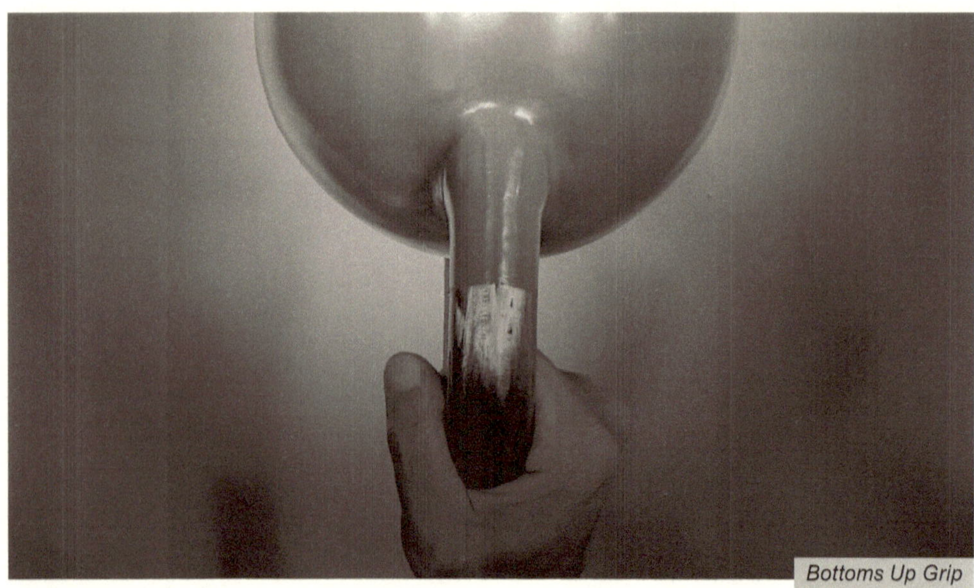

*Bottoms Up Grip*

*Make sure you check out the ebook **Master The Kettlebell Press** which covers all kettlebell presses and is written by yours truly and Joe Daniels.*
*http://bit.ly/2fNV7d1*

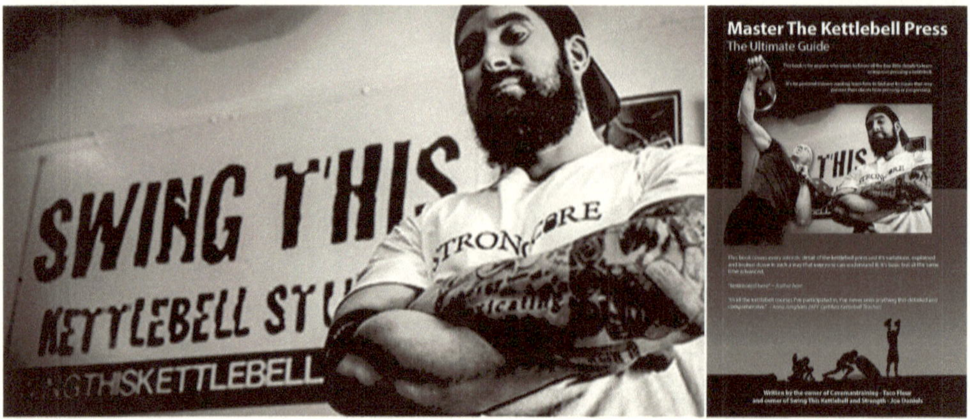

# Horn Grip

**Handle:** two hands, four fingers and thumb locking the index finger down on the horns

**Ideal for:** curls, lunge and twist, halo's

This grip is performed with both hands holding the horns, and is used for doing halo's and bicep curls.

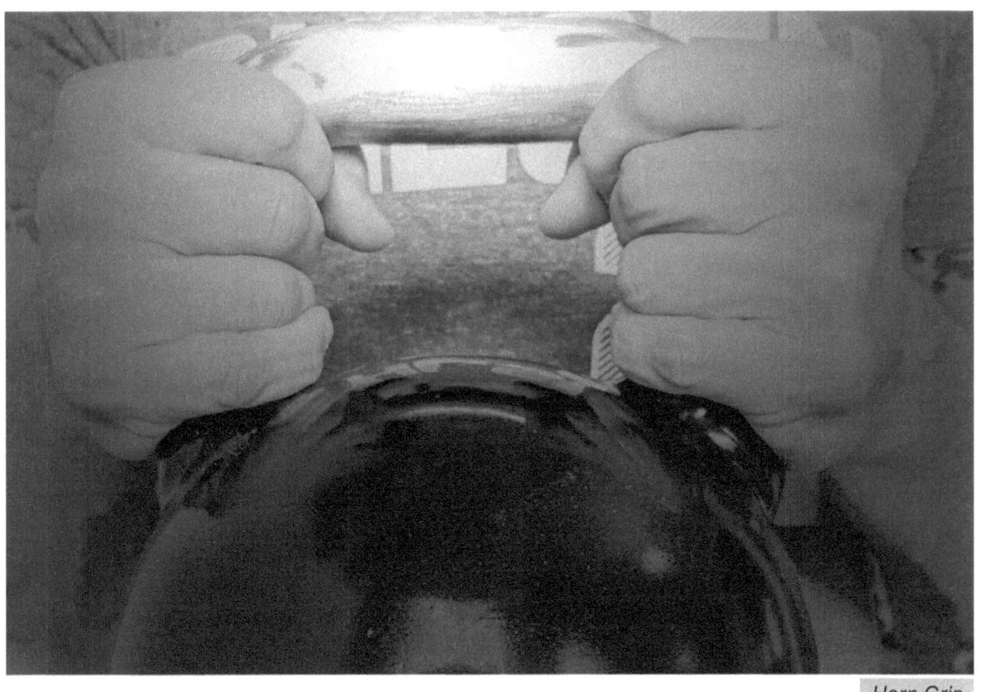

Horn Grip

*Russian twist in action:*
*https://www.youtube.com/watch?v=_KbZno3KZdY*

# Horn Grip Upside Down

**Handle:** two hands, four fingers and thumb locking the index finger down on the horns

**Ideal for:** Russian twists, pull overs, halo's

This grip is performed with the hands holding the horns while the kettlebell is upside down, and can be used for pull-overs and Russian twists.

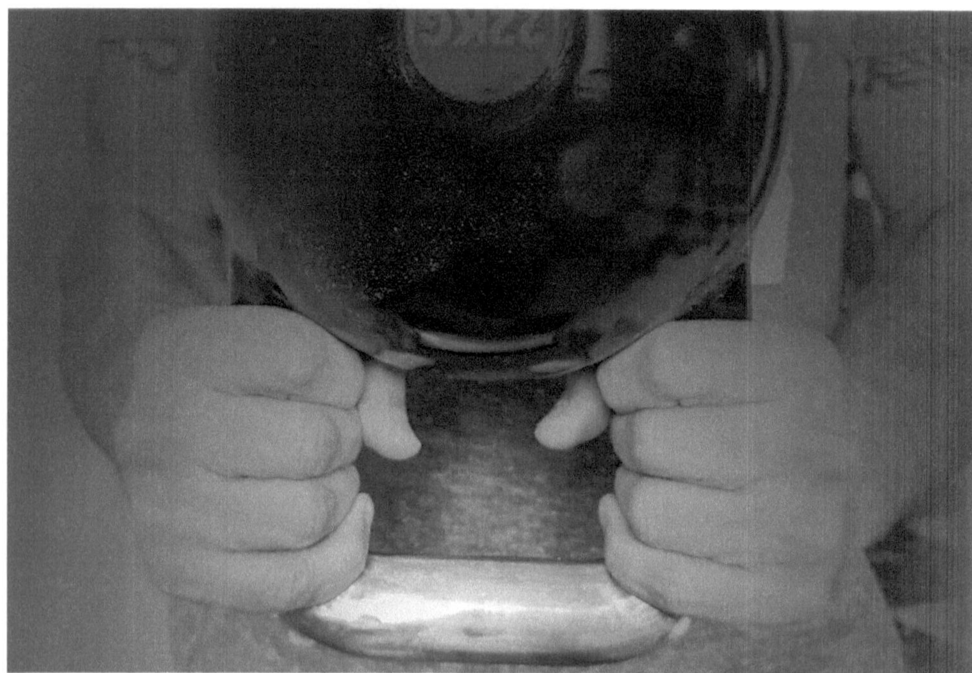

This is also a great grip to work on wrist strength with lateral wrist movement, you can do this in the air with a light bell or have the handle resting on the ground with a heavier bell. When resting the handle on the ground and base is up, the objective is to slowly move the bell forward to where it almost touches the ground, slowly and controlled bringing it back towards you as far as possible.

If you do this drill in the air it also works your biceps as you need to hold the forearms just above horizontal in a static position while moving the wrists. Of course, this will also require you to activate your lats, chest, back and abdominal muscles to provide a solid base where to perform this drill from.

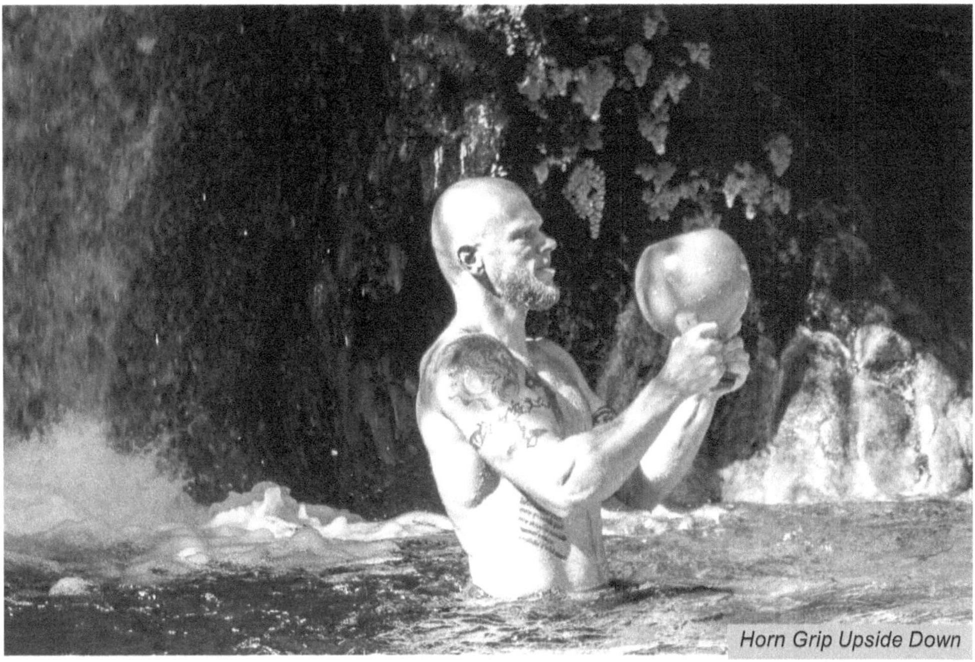

*Horn Grip Upside Down*

*Check out our high quality kettlebell posters and t-shirts that can be purchased online.*

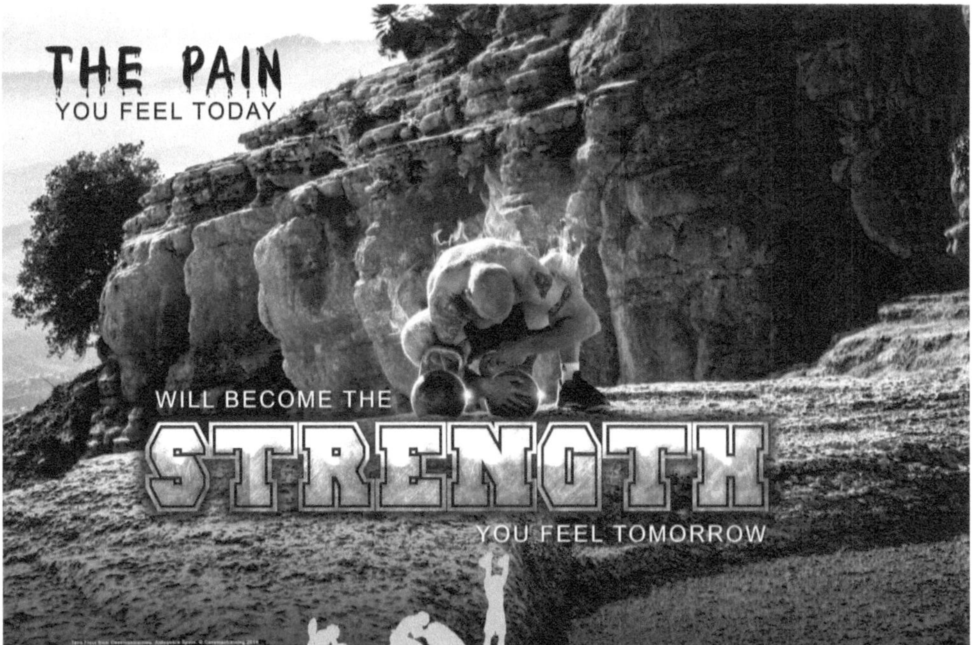

# Corner Grip

**Handle:** one hand, four fingers and thumb loose or locking the index finger down

**Ideal for:** around the body, figure eight.

This grip is performed with the hand holding the handle in the corner, i.e. where the handle and horn intersects, used for around the body and figure eight's. A corner grip is mostly employed for passing the kettlebell to the other hand, whether you're juggling or switching arms.

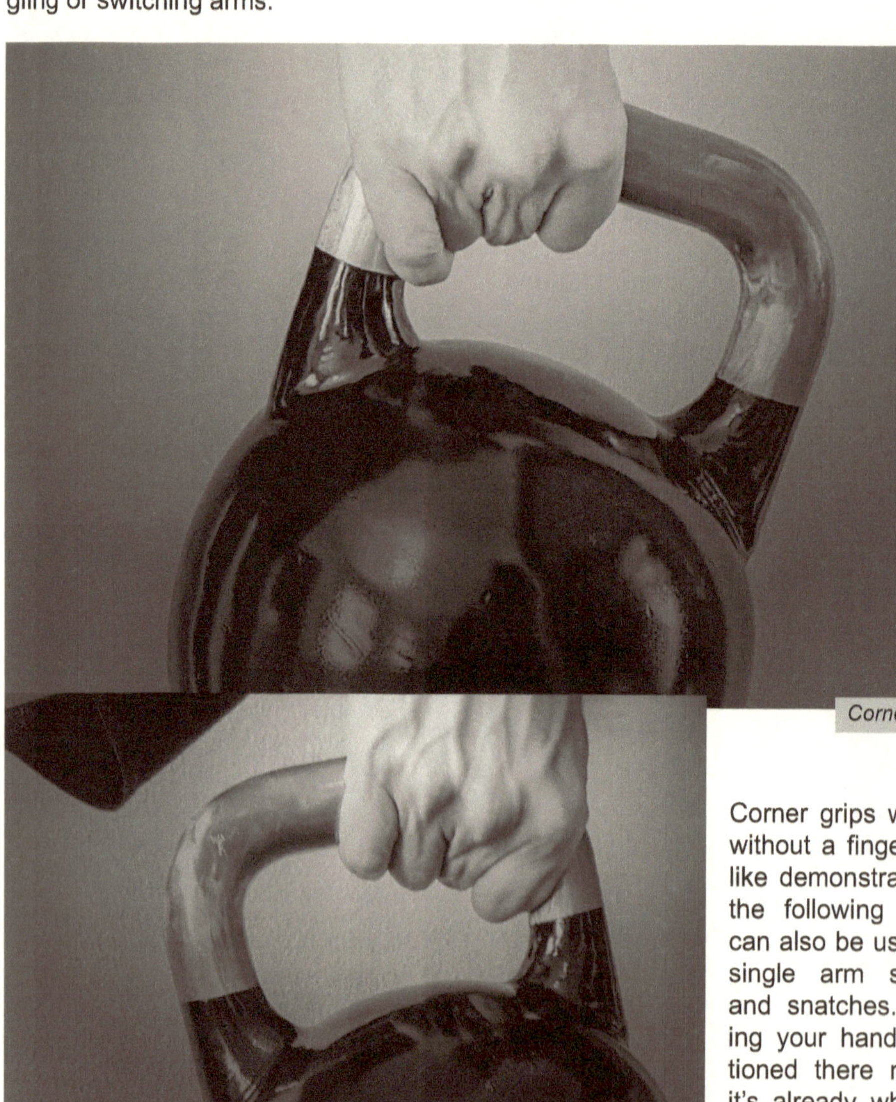

*Corner Grip*

Corner grips with or without a finger lock like demonstrated in the following photo can also be used for single arm swings and snatches. Having your hand positioned there means it's already where it needs to end up in overhead position.

# Open Hand Horn Grip

**Handle:** two hands, all fingers slightly squeezing the bell and the thumbs folded around the bottom of the horns

**Ideal for:** laying down chest presses, front squats, skull crushers.

With this grip both hands are used, palms are open and slightly squeezing the bell which is resting within the palms, the thumbs are folded around the bottom of the horns. This grip is used for front squats and skull crushers.

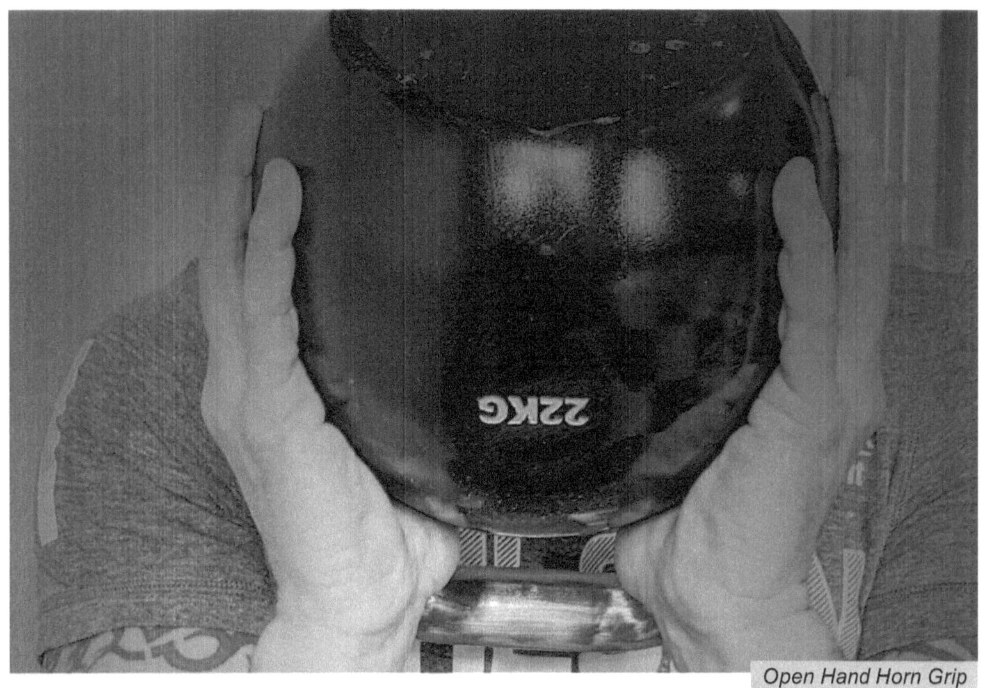

*Open Hand Horn Grip*

# Loose Grip

**Handle:** one hand, four fingers and thumb loosely around the handle

**Ideal for:** any press variation, any overhead work, racking

This grip is performed by keeping your fingers loose rather than tightly closed and squeezing, it's used for the overhead position like presses and snatches.

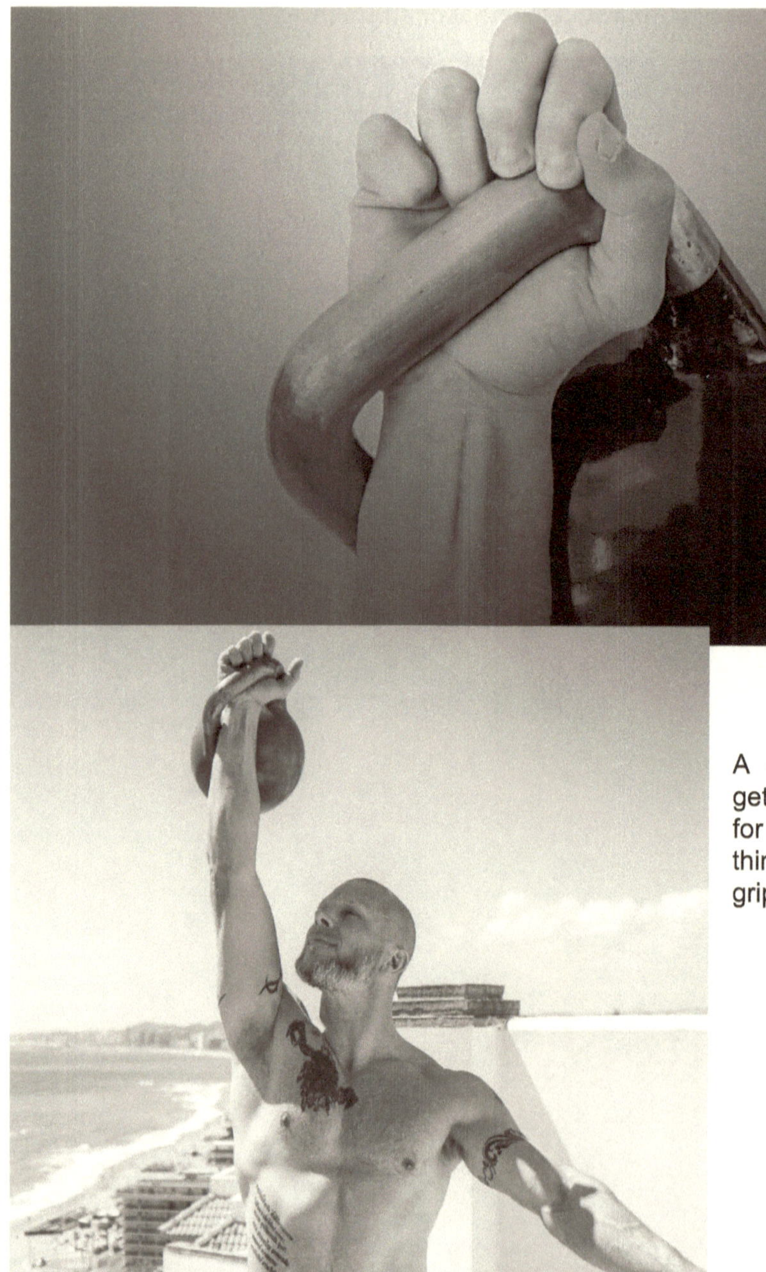

*Loose Grip*

A great analogy to get the idea across for CrossFitters is thinking about a false grip.

# Interlocking Grip

**Handle:** two hands, all fingers interlocking and thumb through the corners

**Ideal for:** racking rest, anything performed with a rack, front squats.

This grip is performed by interlocking the fingers of both hands, elbows tight into the side of the body, and is used for front squats or racked lunges.

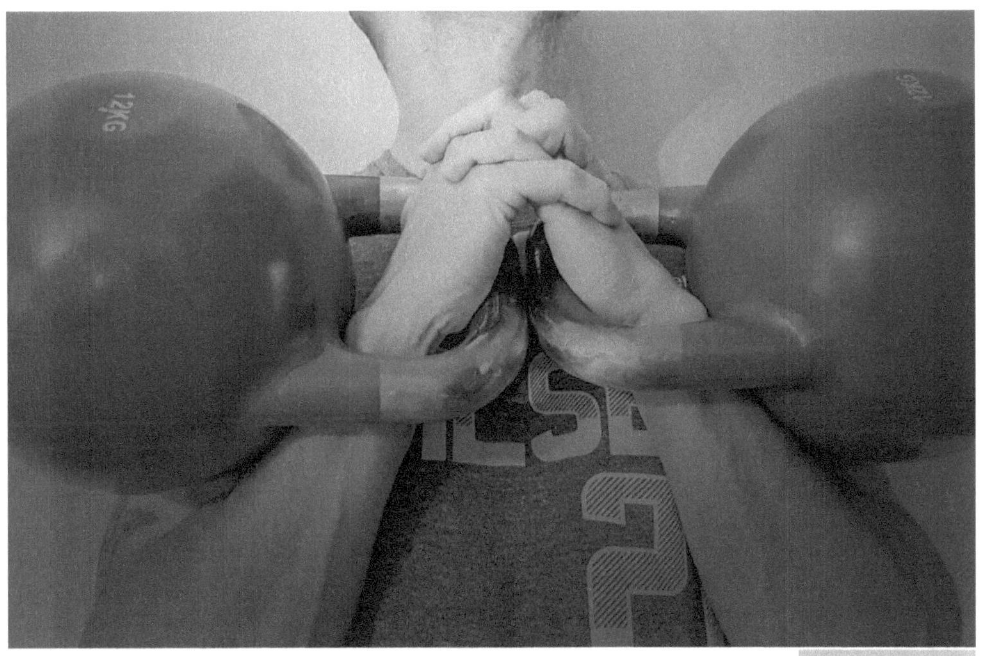

*Interlocking Grip*

# Stacking Grip

**Handle:** two hands, several fingers holding on to the handle of the stacked kettlebell

**Ideal for:** racking rest, anything going rack to overhead.

This grip is performed by placing the handles on top of each other and several fingers holding on to the second handle while the top hand is over the bottom hand, used for resting or anything going overhead like the press, push press or jerk.

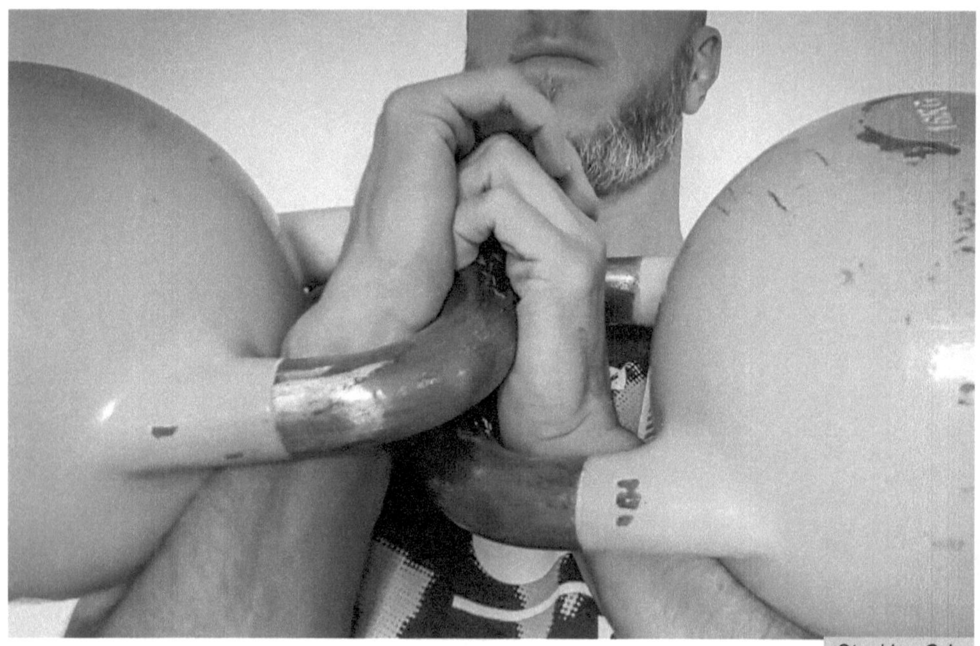

*Stacking Grip*

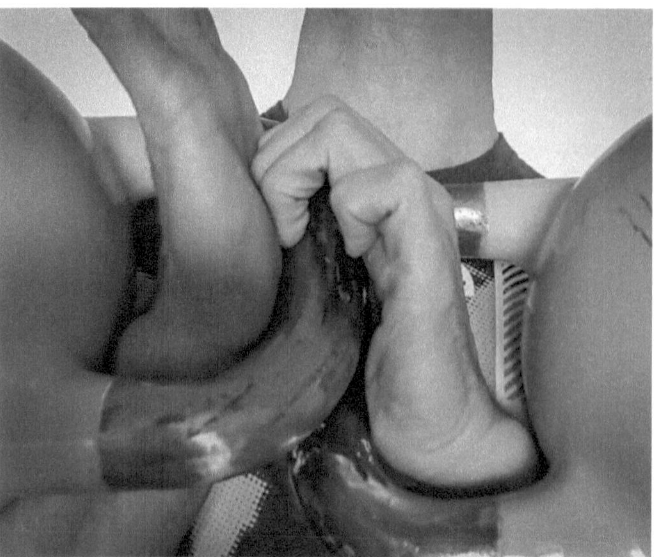

Illustrated is the bottom hand and the area the fingers grip on the top handle

# Open Palm Grip

**Handle:** handle is resting against the underside of the forearm

**Ideal for:** increasing difficulty of presses.

This grip is performed with the bell resting in the open palm and handle against the underside of the forearm. Great for working on wrist strength.

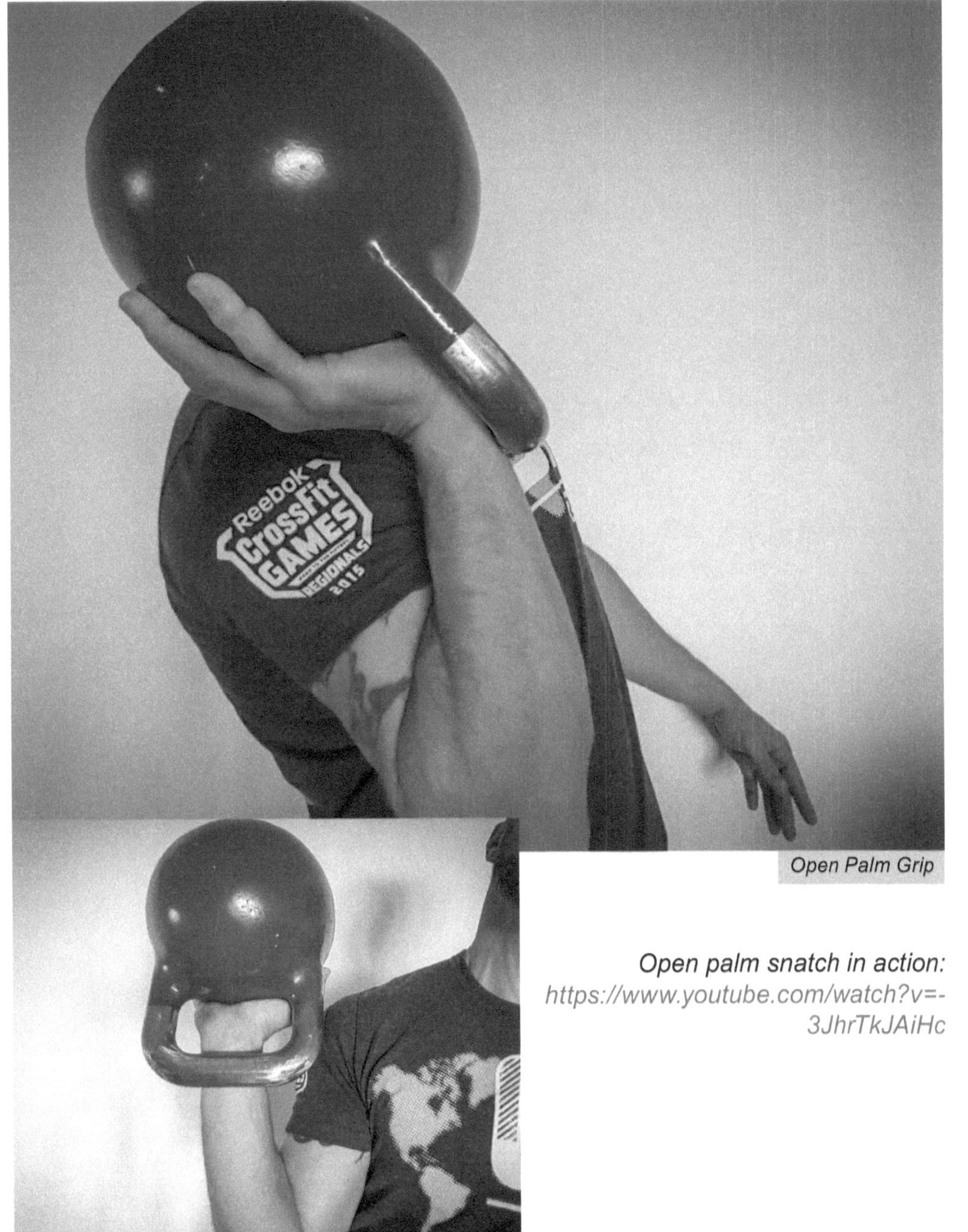

Open Palm Grip

*Open palm snatch in action:*
*https://www.youtube.com/watch?v=-*
*3JhrTkJAiHc*

# Waiters Grip

Handle: the handle does not come into play

**Ideal for:** increasing difficulty of presses.

This grip is performed with the base resting on the open palm.  Great for working on wrist strength. This grip is named for obvious reasons, the way the kettlebell rests on the palm resembles that of a waiter carrying a tray.

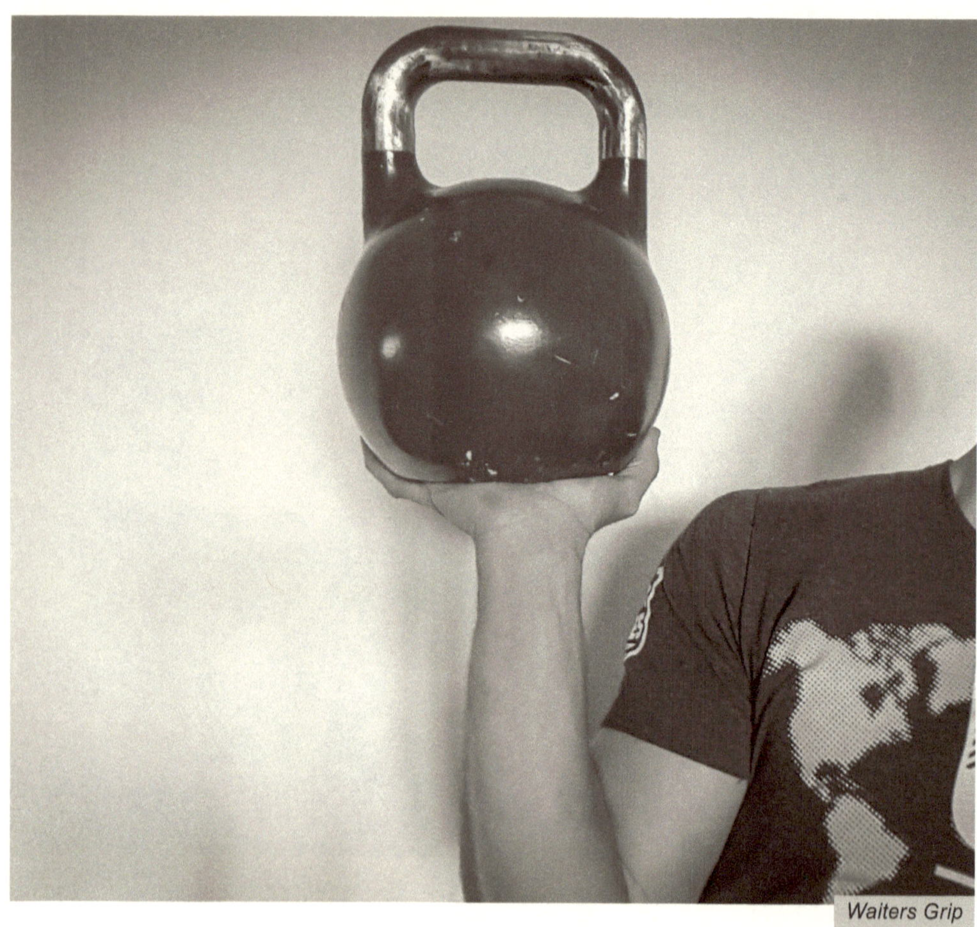

*Waiters Grip*

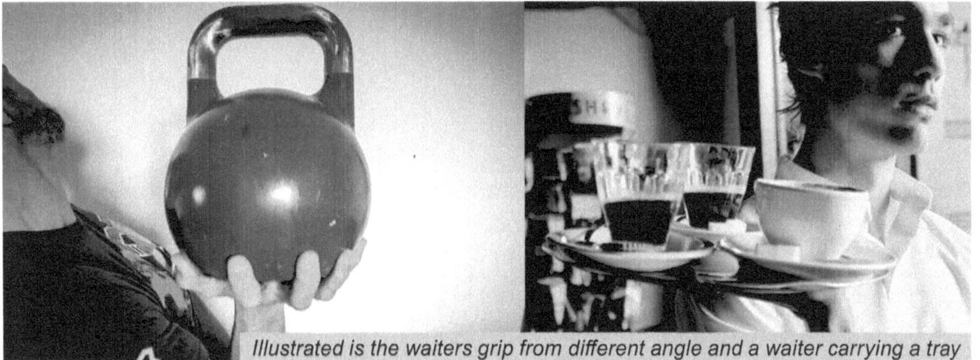

*Illustrated is the waiters grip from different angle and a waiter carrying a tray*

Once you get into kettlebell juggling you can swing and catch the kettlebell directly into waiters grip, from there you can perform an overhead squat. This variation requires a more explosive swing to get the kettlebell high and flip into waiters grip.

*You can see the waiters grip in action here: https://www.youtube.com/watch?v=s9ZP5_mWFws*

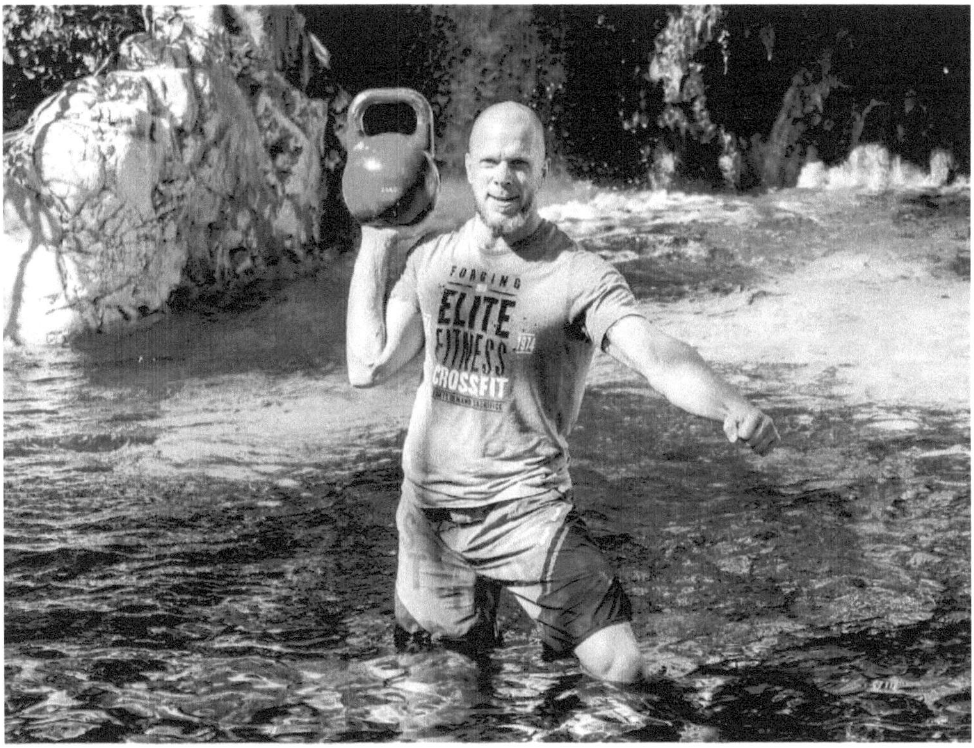

*I'm always available to answer any question you might have, add me on facebook*
*www.facebook.com/taco.fleur **or here** www.facebook.com/coach.taco.fleur/*

# Goblet Grip

**Handle:** the handle does not come into play

**Ideal for:** front-squat.

This grip is performed with the palms pressing around the bell, the handle is up or down. The grip is named for obvious reasons, the shape of the kettlebell with handle down resembles that of a goblet. With the handle facing up this grip is called the reverse goblet grip. The higher you go up the bell with your palms, the harder you need to squeeze, palms towards the bottom and the bell is resting more within the palms.

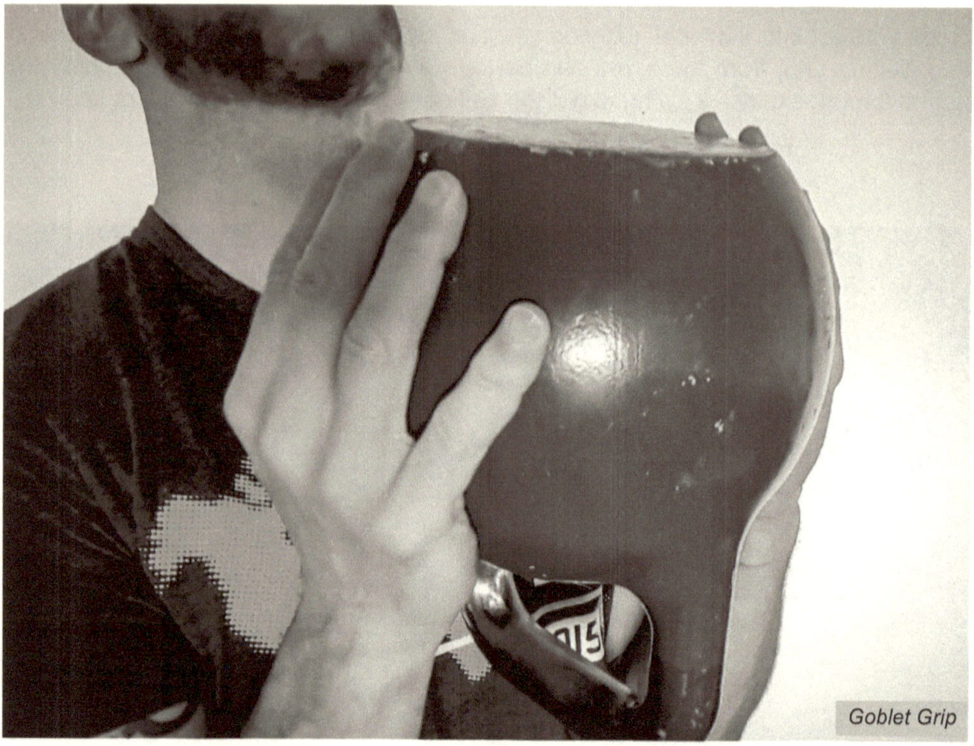

*Goblet Grip*

*There is a lot of confusion about the goblet grip and for that reason I wrote an article which I recommend reading www.cavemantraining.com/caveman-kettlebells/goblet-squat-rather-goblet-grip/*

*You can watch a video demonstrating the goblet grip in a goblet squat. www.youtube.com/watch?v=peuGSnbgXEk*

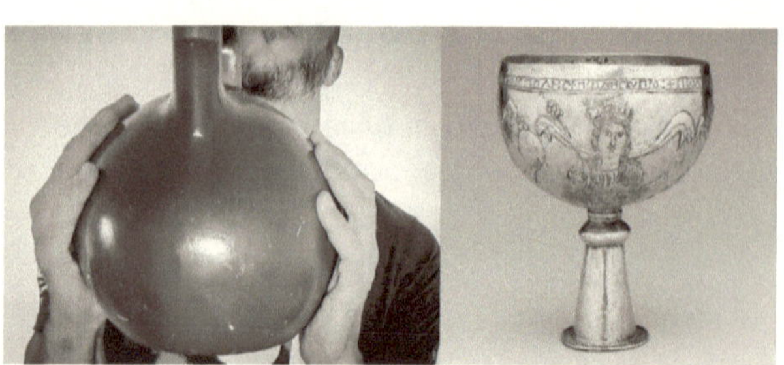

*Illustrated is the reverse goblet grip and a golden goblet*

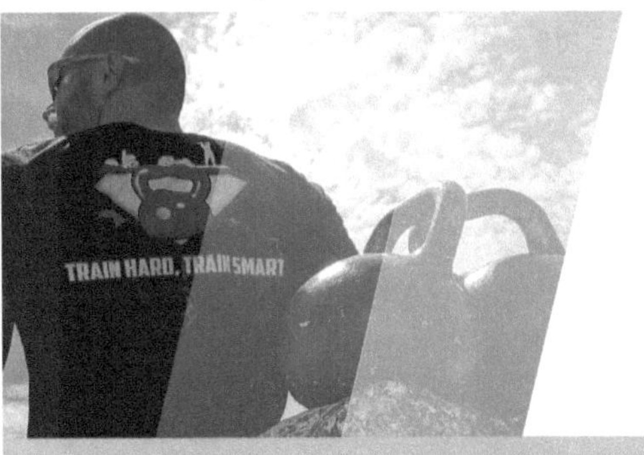
TRAIN HARD, TRAIN SMART
KETTLEBELL TRAINING FUNDAMENTALS
FROM ZERO TO KETTLEBELL SUPERHERO
Check out
our high quality
kettlebell posters
and t-shirts
that can be pur-
chased online.

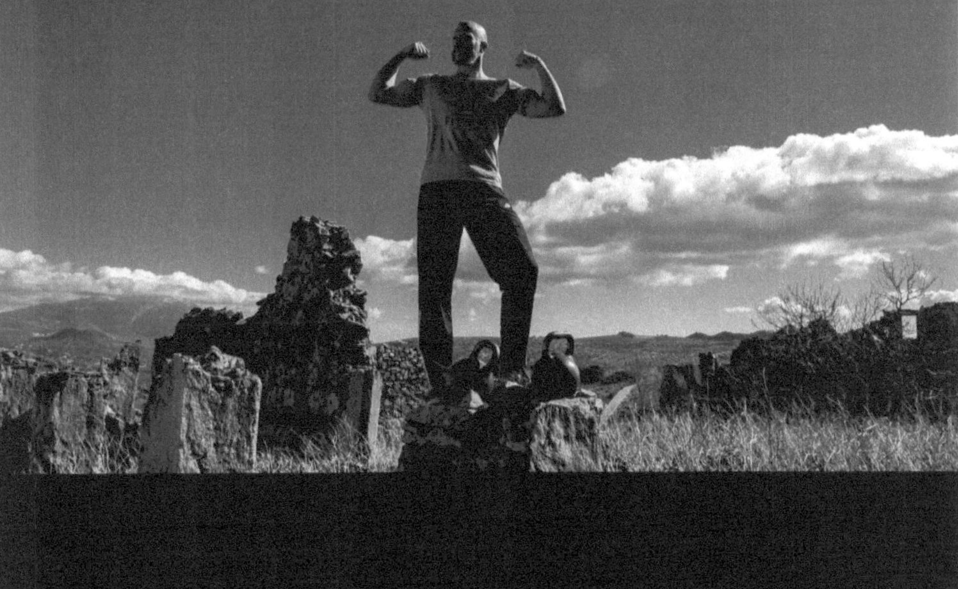
"Don't work 8 hours for a company then go home and not work
on your own goals. You're not tired, you're uninspired."

# Crush Grip

**Handle:** the handle does not come into play

**Ideal for:** front-squat, static hold, push-up.

This grip is performed with the palms crushing the bell, the handle is up or down. Similar to the goblet grip but more crushing with the palms. Great for working the pectoralis.

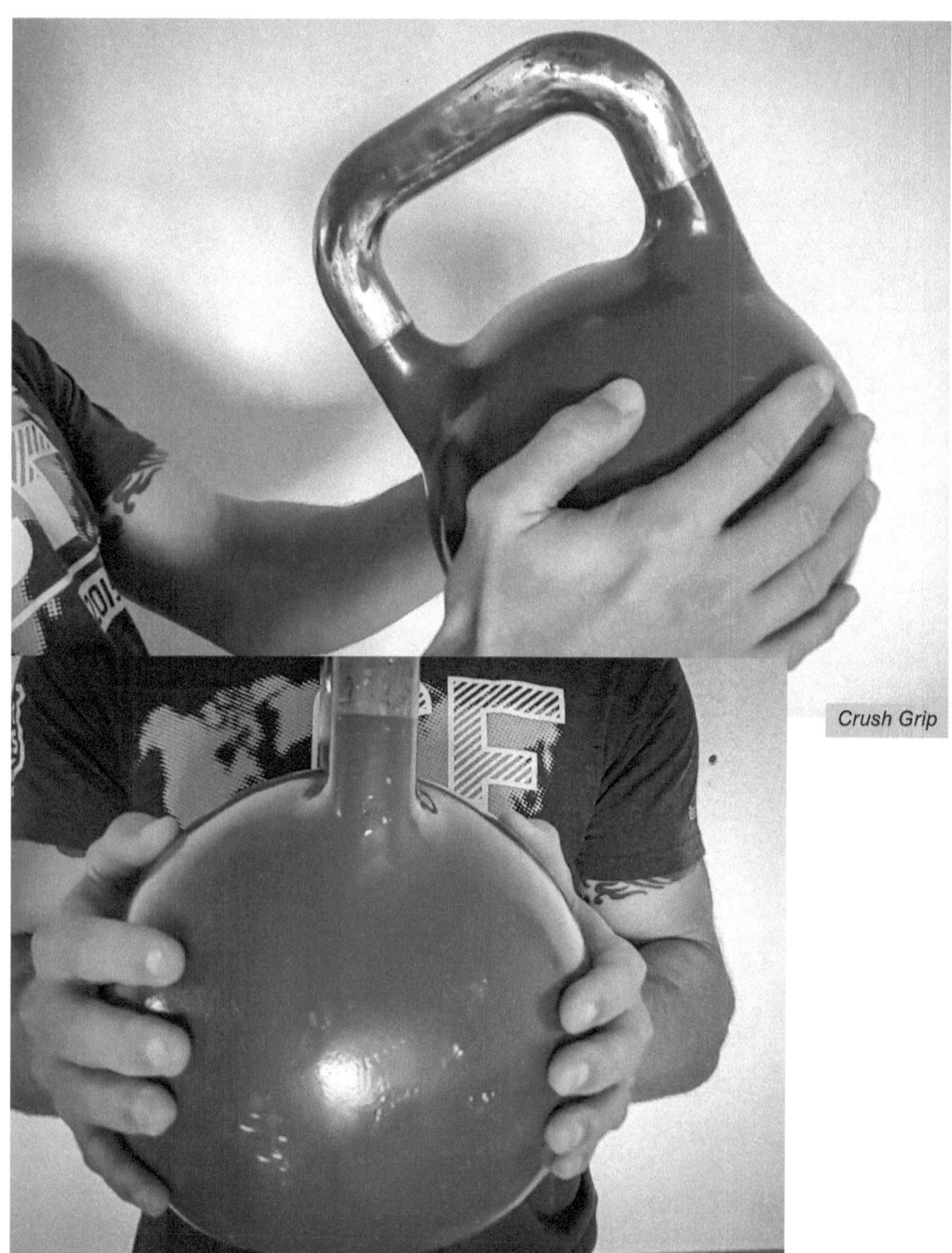

Crush Grip

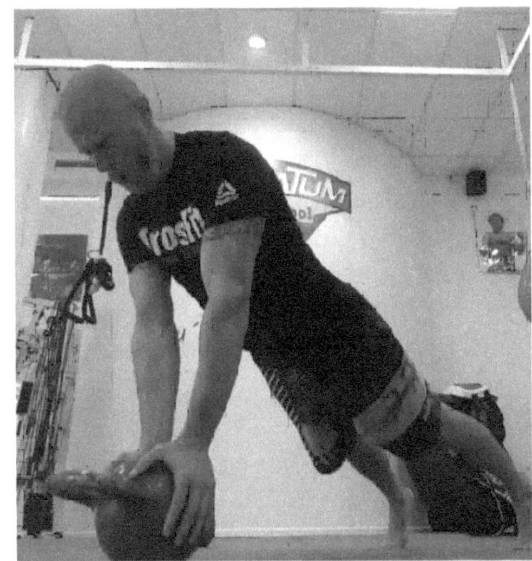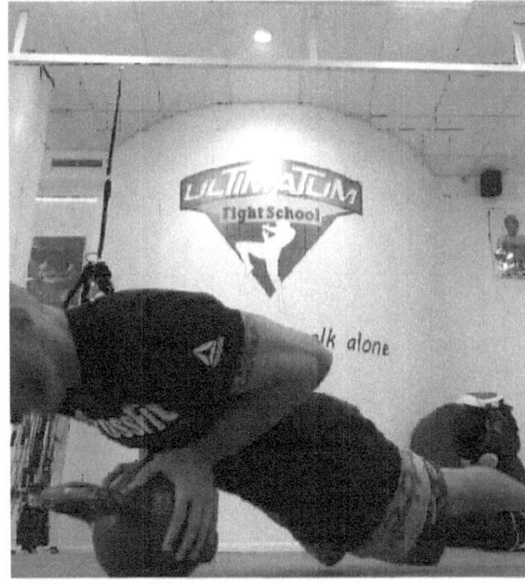

*Have you tried the kettlebell crush push-up yet?*

*You can also watch a short video here:*
www.instagram.com/p/BZs28yhB4WH/

*High quality kettlebell and unique posters can be purchased online*

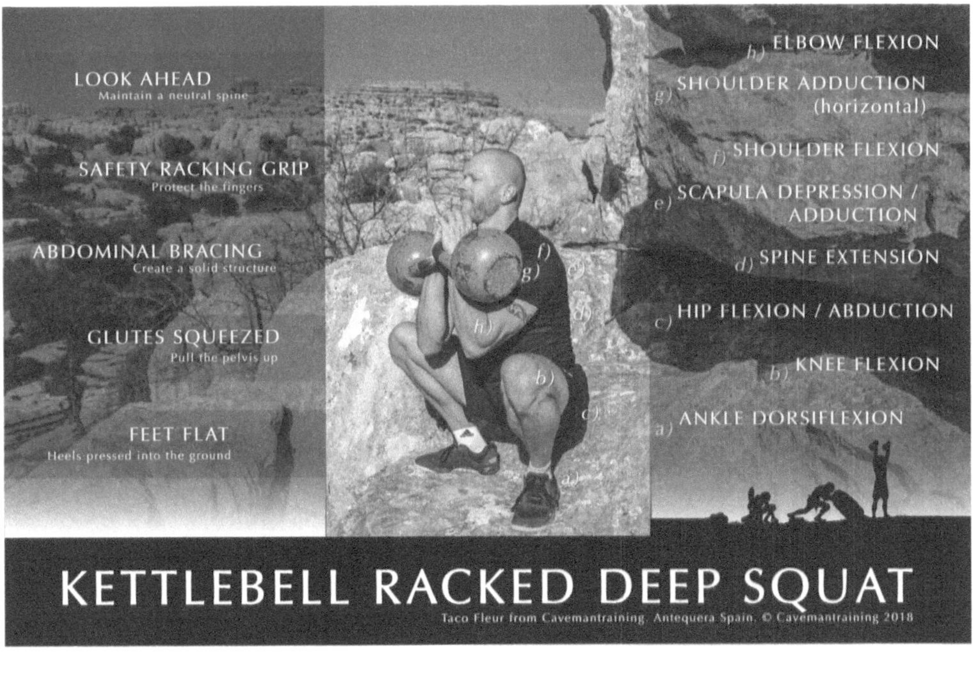

# Thumb Grip (AKA Noob Grip)

**Handle:** the handle is resting more on the heel of the thumb than with the loose grip.

**Ideal for:** press.

The bell rests on the inside of the arm, complete opposite of the loose grip, the handle is resting more on the heel of the thumb. Great for shifting the weight from the outside of the arm to the inside. Full range reps from racking are not possible with this grip. Try this one with the side press starting above the shoulder and returning above the shoulder.

I like to call this the noob grip as this is the grip a lot of new people use the first ever time they lift a kettlebell without instruction.

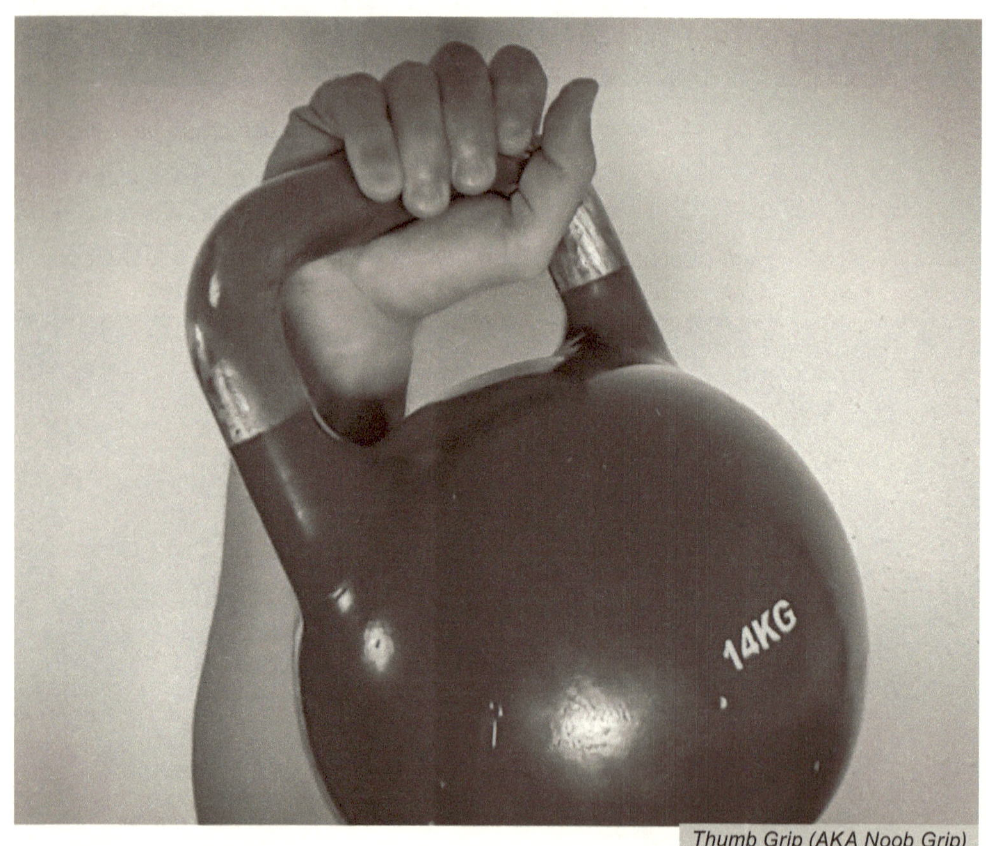

*Thumb Grip (AKA Noob Grip)*

*Find out why I named this the noob grip
and why it's such a great grip to employ after you learned all other grips.*
*www.cavemantraining.com/caveman-kettlebells/
24-unconventional-kettlebell-exercises-three-broken/*

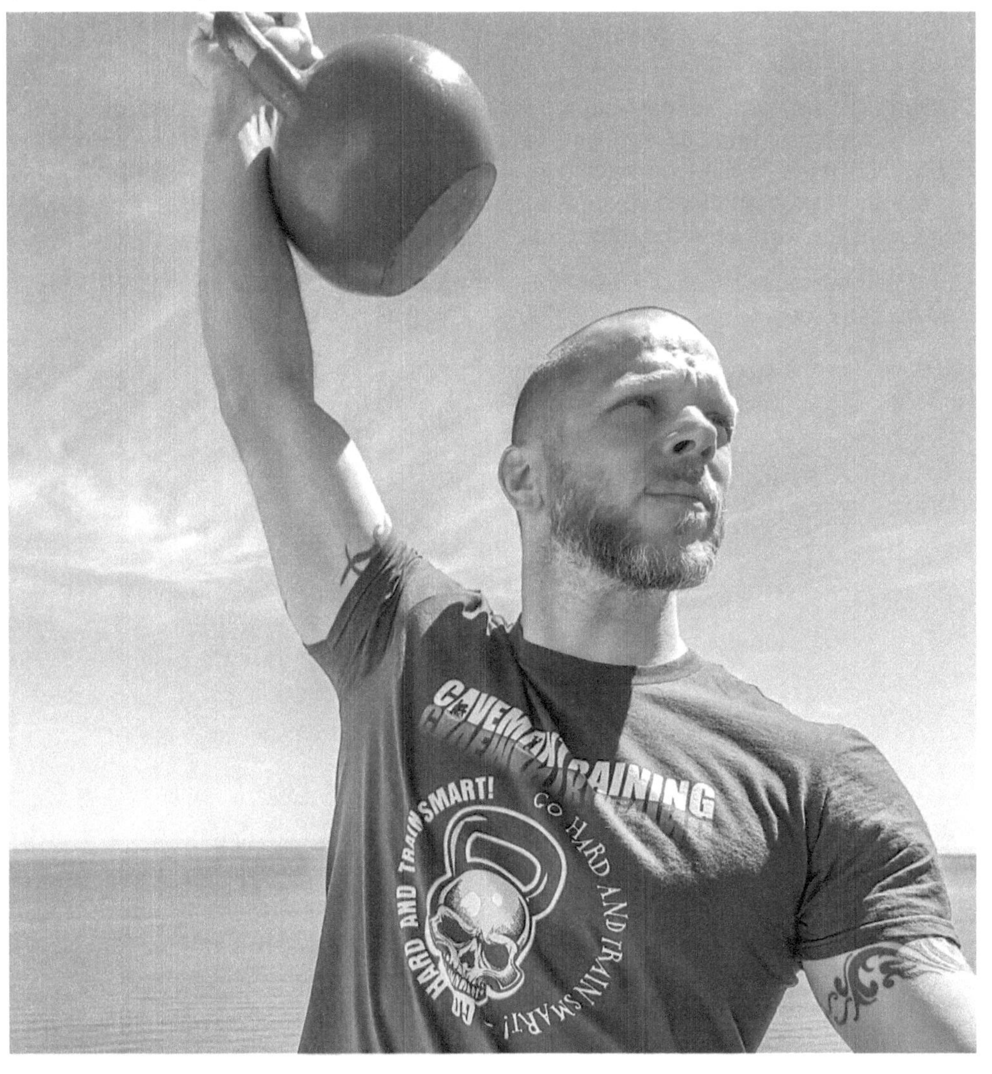

*More info about the noob grip squat can be found here*
www.cavemantraining.com/caveman-kettlebells/even-kettlebell-squat-bro/


*Check out the combination of noob grip squat and press, try it yourself
and notice the instability it provides, which is great once you've gained some strength
and technique by implementing common grips.*
www.youtube.com/watch?v=Q8t05MbK_R4

# Fireman's Grip

This grip is solely used for carrying the kettlebells on or over the shoulders and is what I call the fireman's grip due to the close resemblance of the fireman's carry. With this grip your hand is holding the handle in the middle and is resting more in the fingers, the elbows are up and the kettlebell is resting on or over your shoulder. Can be performed with one or two kettlebells, one on each side.

Great for back squats, i.e. the weight is resting on the back rather than the front, can also be used for just carrying the kettlebells and walking.

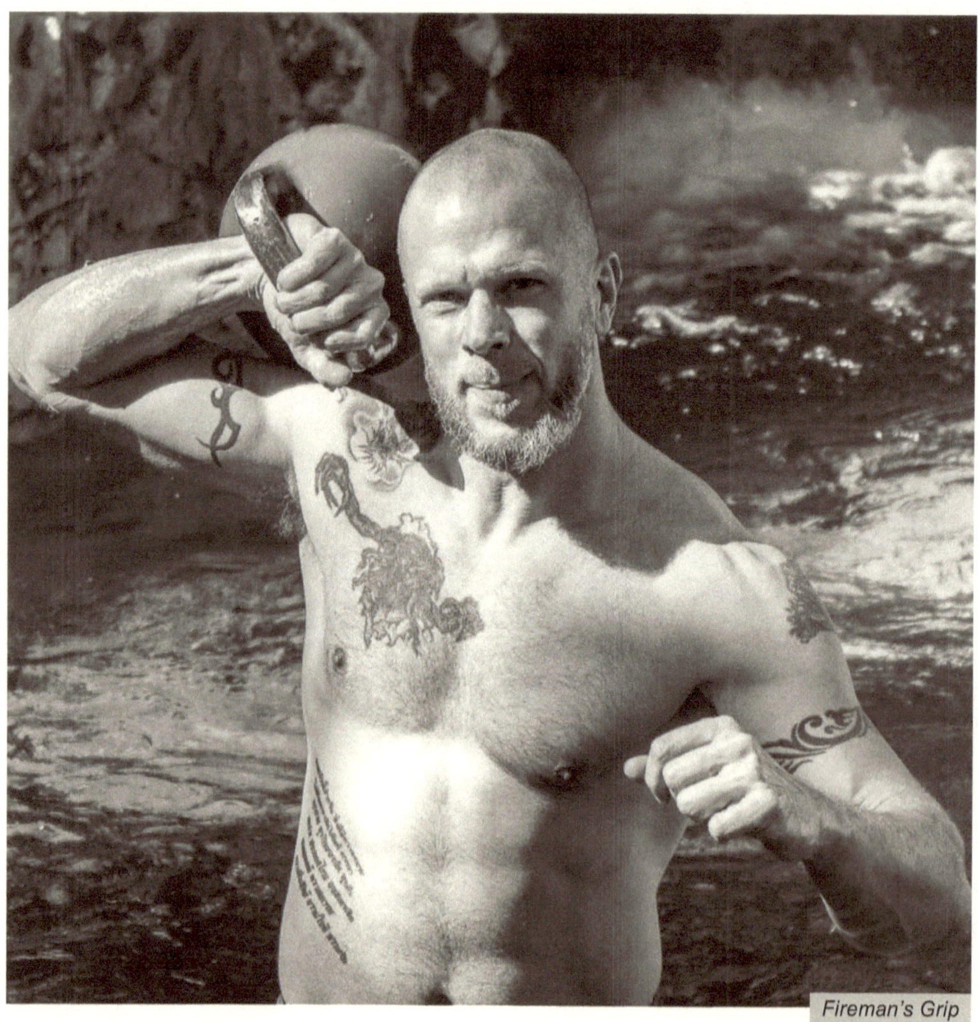

*Fireman's Grip*

*Watch a demonstration of the Fireman's Squat in the following video*
*https://www.youtube.com/watch?v=PG1dm0MJD4o*

# Stacked Grip

This grip is used to work with multiple kettlebells in one hand. It's a great grip to add more weight to your deadlifts or overhead work. The grip requires a lot more grip strength as well, as double or triple handles/weight will require more grip strength.

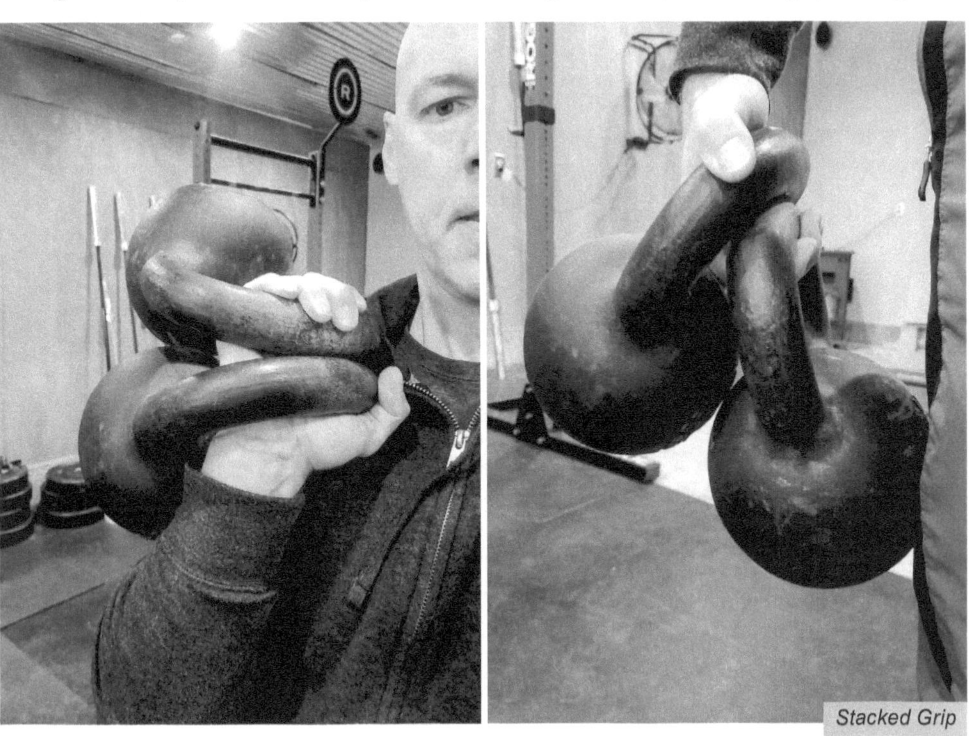

Stacked Grip

*Photo provided by Robert Gagnon SFG II*
*www.RobGagnon.com*

# NOTE

If you experience forearm bruising, tenderness or pain from bell pressure, make sure you check out my detailed article on this topic, you won't find anything more detailed and intricate about this issue elsewhere. Search Google for 'Caveman-training forearm pressure, bruising and pain'.

If you're after more detailed instructions or want to know more about kettlebell pressing, check out our book *Master The Kettlebell Press*, it covers a lot of details on the press, including some fine tuning to avoid injuries etc.

"Taco Fleur and Joe Daniels have hit the nail on the head with this book. This is the ONLY guide you'll ever need if you are into Kettlebell Training or CrossFit." ~ *Don Giafardino*

"Over 100 kettlebell press variations in one book is pretty impressive!" ~ *Anna Junghans (IKFF Certified Kettlebell Teacher)*

"Taco Fleur and Joe Daniels are honest, humble and direct with their instruction in Master the Kettlebell Press. A must read for anyone that incorporates kettlebells into their training. Whether a novice or professional; you'll appreciate the value in the content of this book."
~ *Kelly Manzone (Kettlebell Sport Athlete)*

**cavemantraining.com/kettlebell-press**

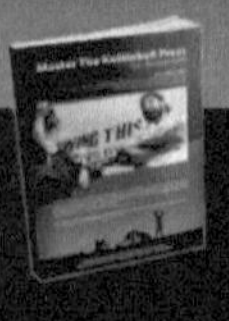
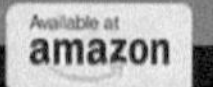
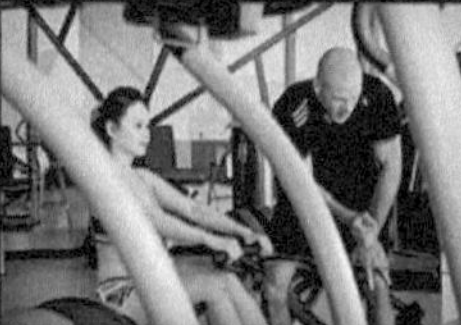
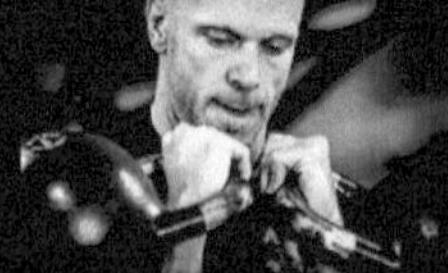
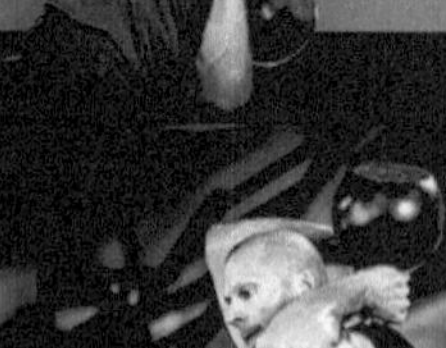

Also available on Amazon in kindle and print version
amazon.com/Master-Kettlebell-Press-Ultimate-Training-ebook/dp/B01N4ORE-OW/

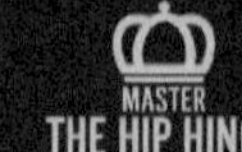

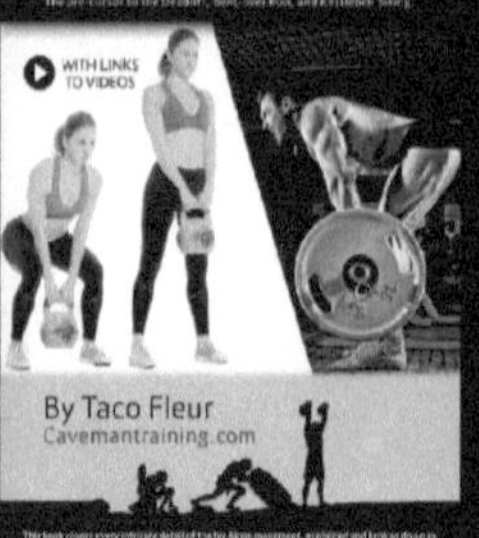


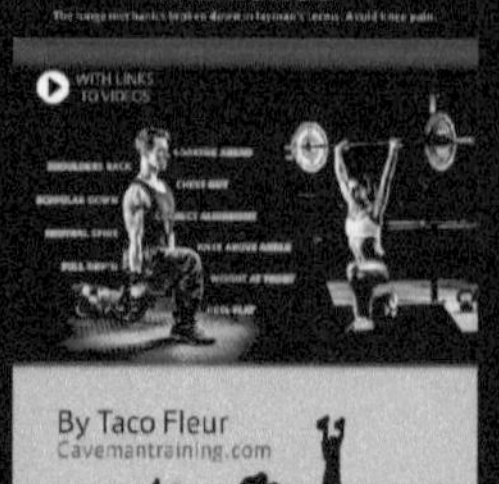


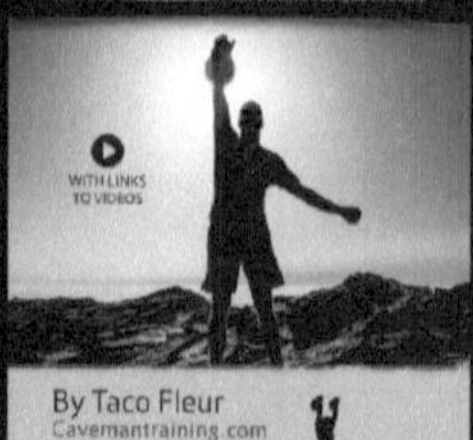

*All images are copyright Cavemantraining*

*Kettlebell stock images are available for purchase or in some cases made available for educational purpose with appropriate credits/links.*

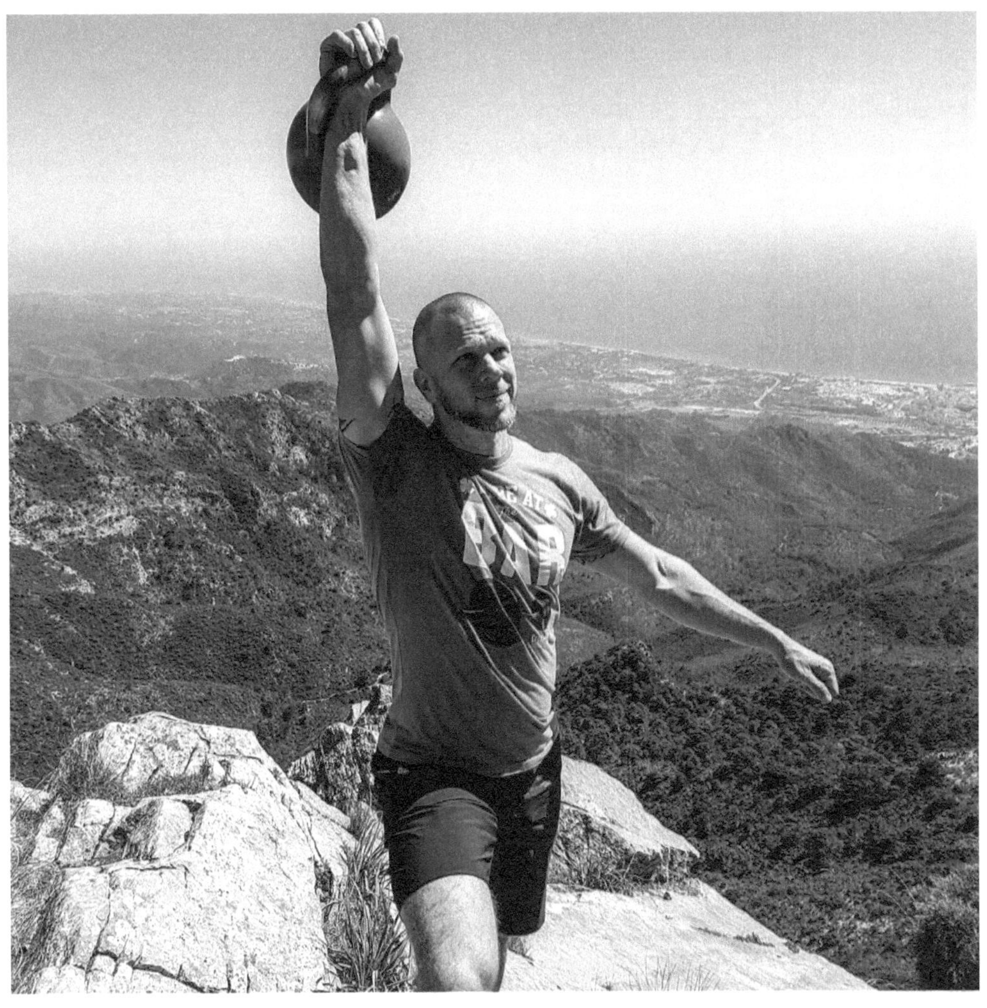

*If you enjoyed the content of this book, please take a few seconds of your time and consider leaving a review or post on our Facebook page. Thanks.*

*www.facebook.com/pg/caveman.training/reviews/*

*I'm always available to answer any question you might have, add me on facebook www.facebook.com/taco.fleur or here www.facebook.com/coach.taco.fleur/*

*Check out the free kettlebell videos from Cavemantraining on Youtube*
*youtube.com/channel/UCBRIDOmwDoptO7LrdlUhs0g*


*Check out this awesome resource for kettlebell training*
*www.cavemantraining.com/caveman-kettlebells/what-is-kettlebell-training/*


*Created with the help of Anna Junghans.*

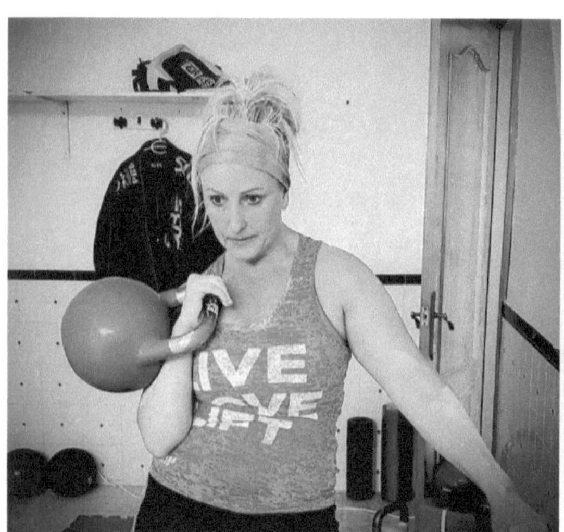

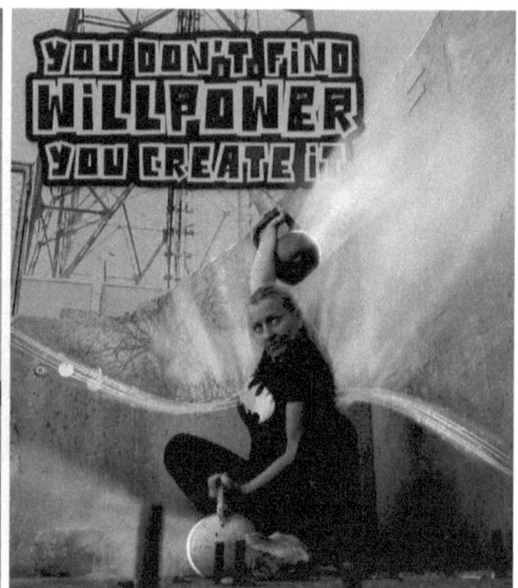

Created by Taco Fleur
Copyright 2018

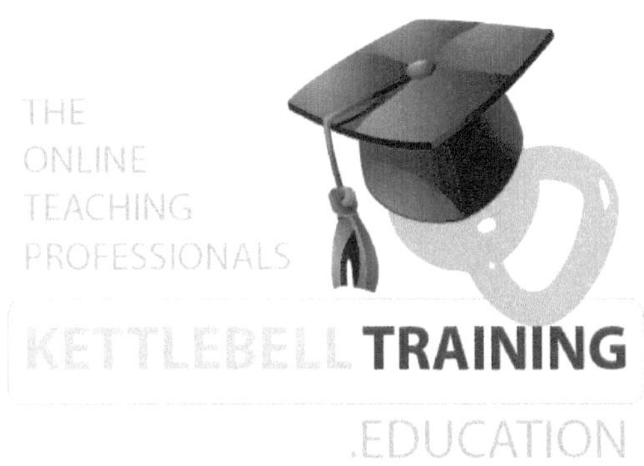

kettlebelltraining.education

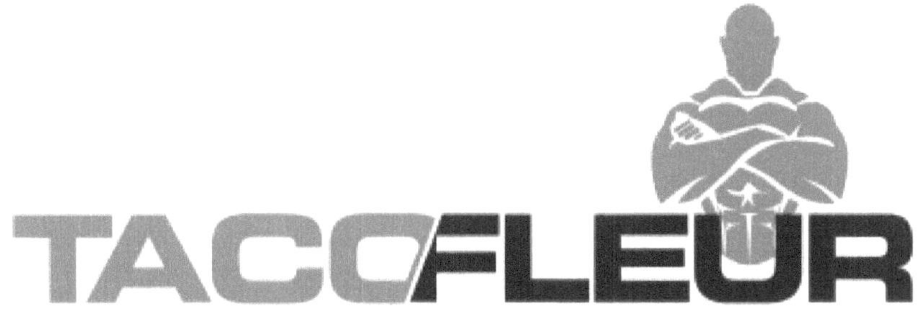

www.tacofleur.com

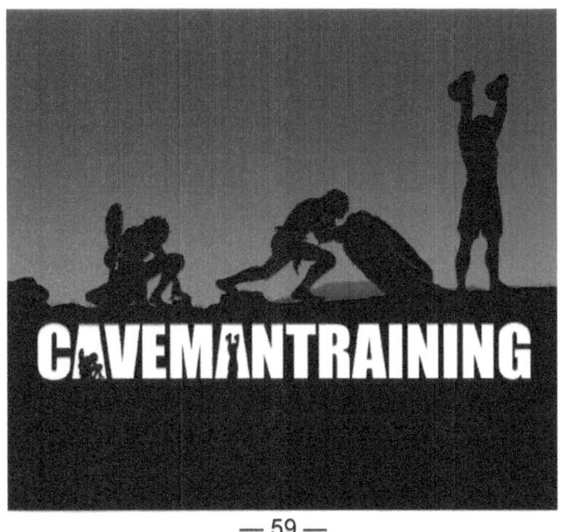

www.ingramcontent.com/pod-product-compliance
Lightning Source LLC
Chambersburg PA
CBHW051235250726

48655CB00006B/2792